Heavy Metal Toxicity in Public Health

Edited by John Kanayochukwu Nduka and Mohamed Nageeb Rashed

Published in London, United Kingdom

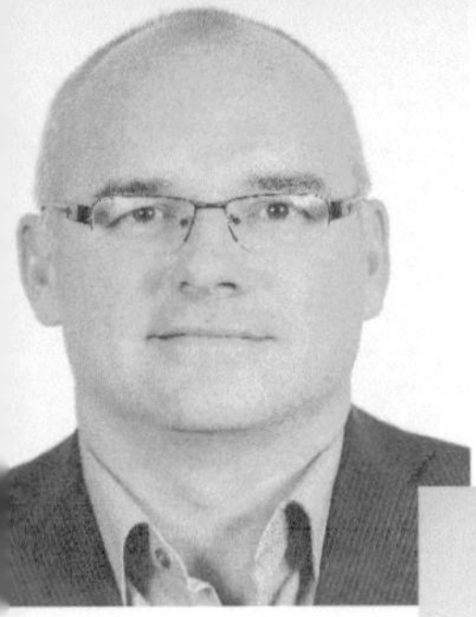
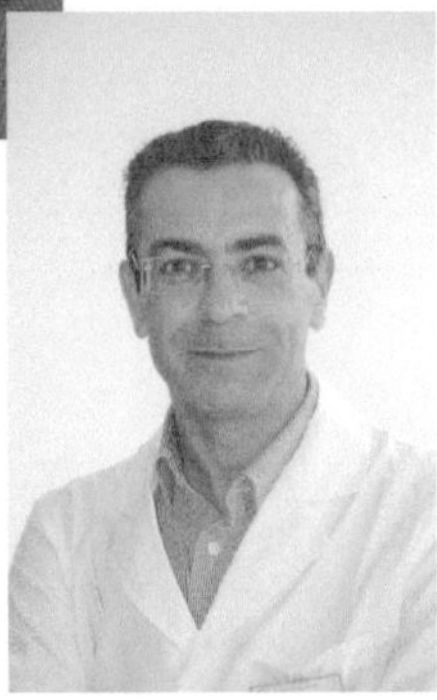
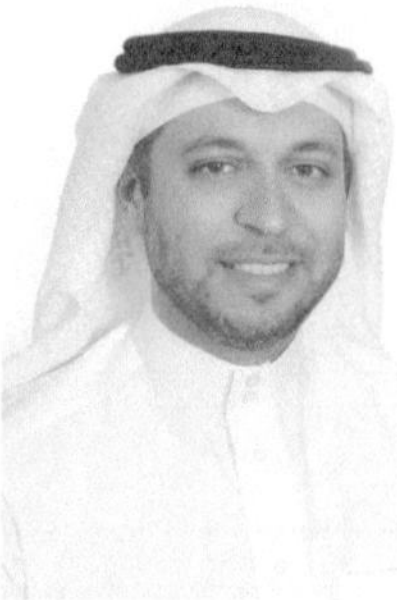
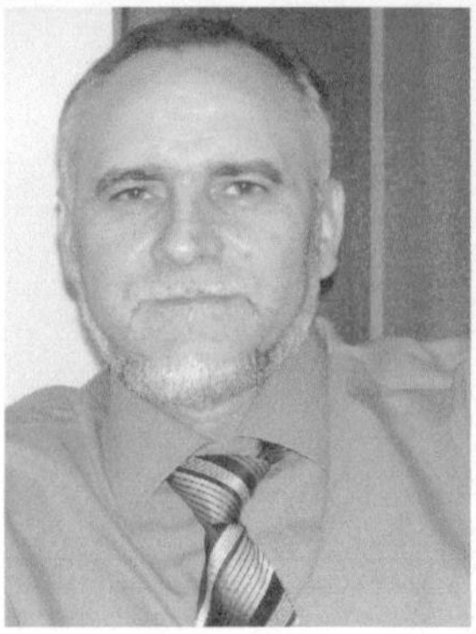
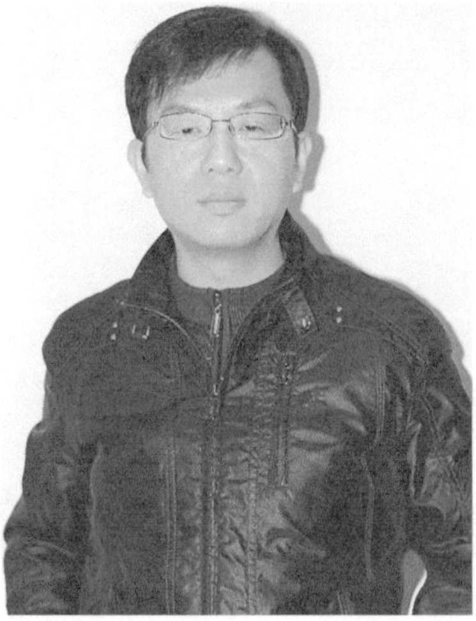
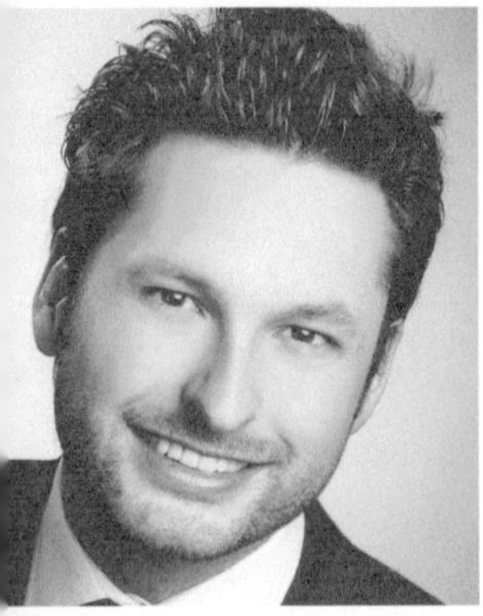
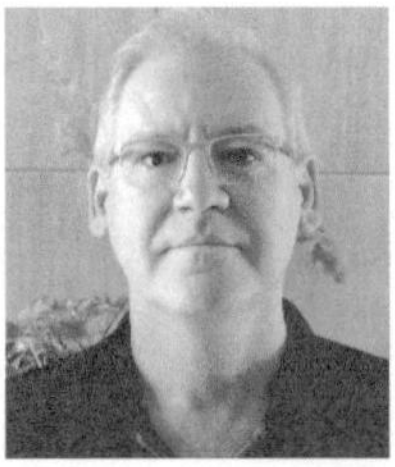

IntechOpen

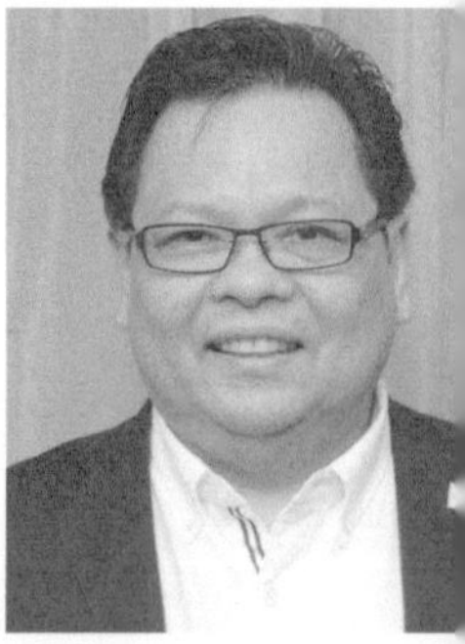
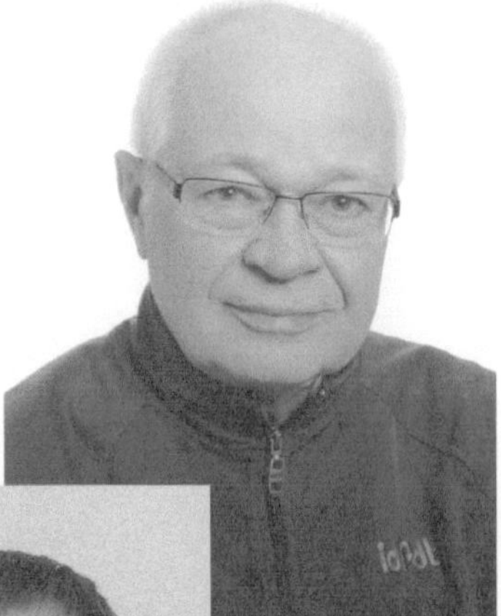
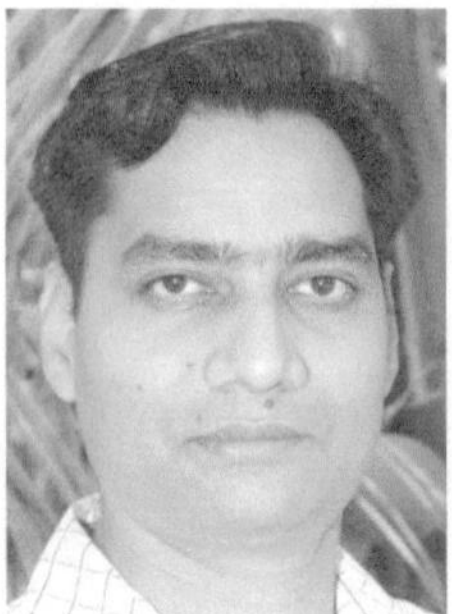
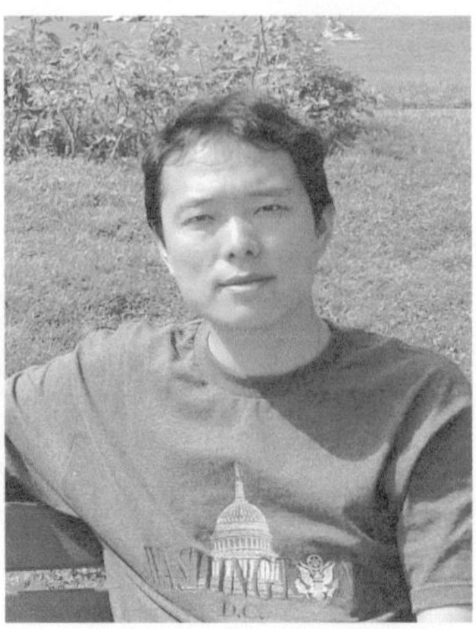
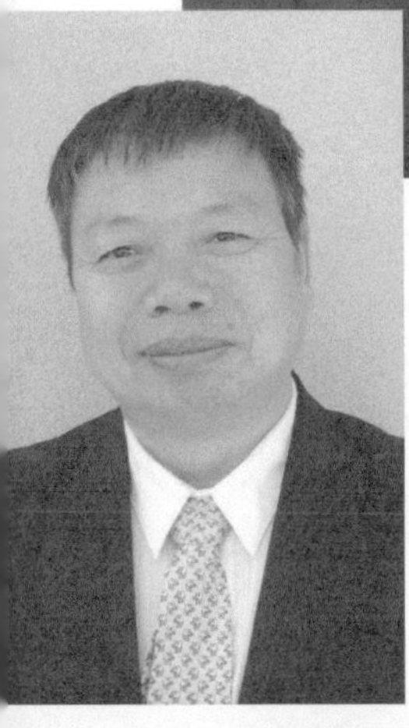
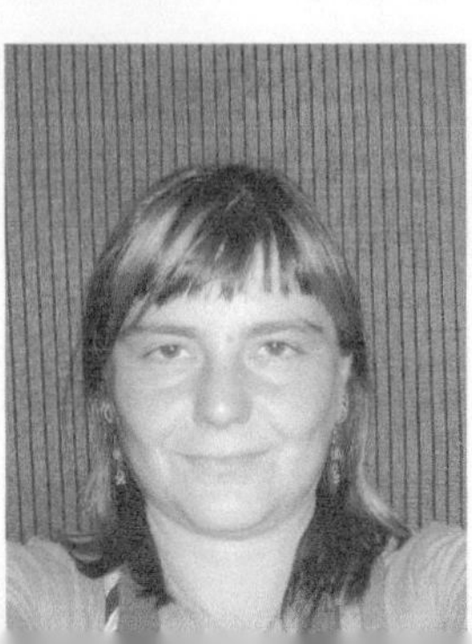

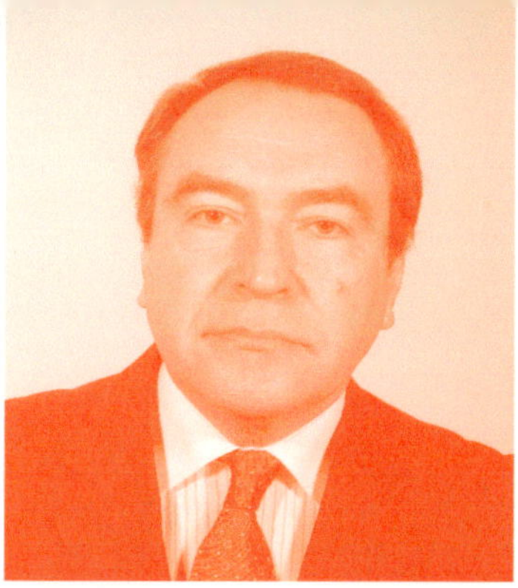

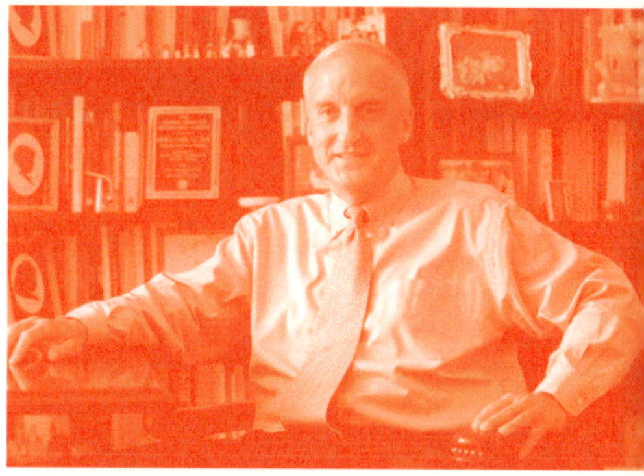

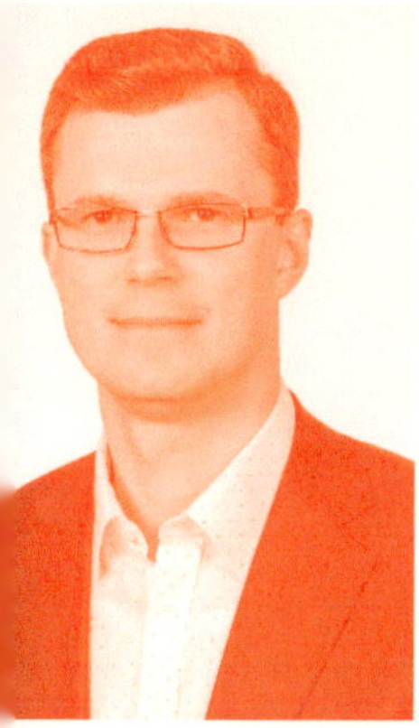

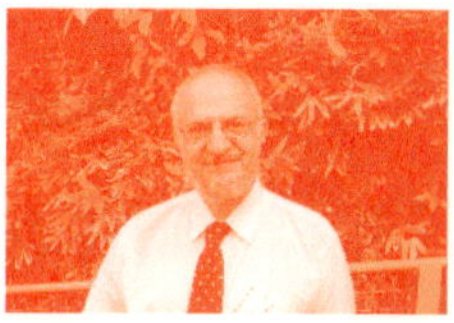

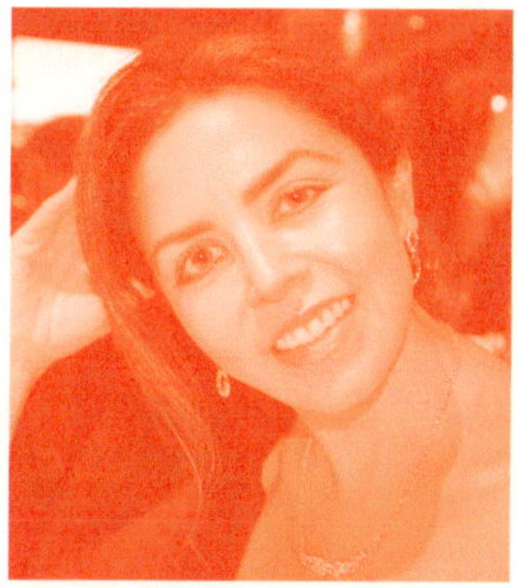

Supporting open minds since 2005

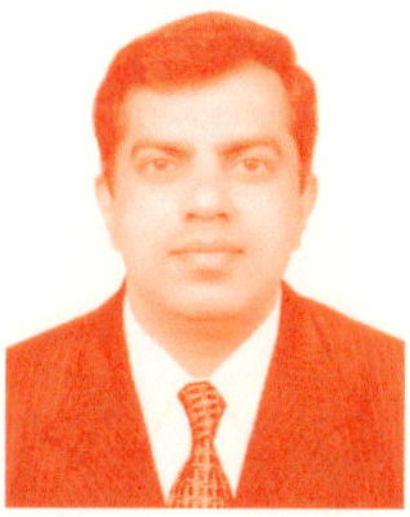

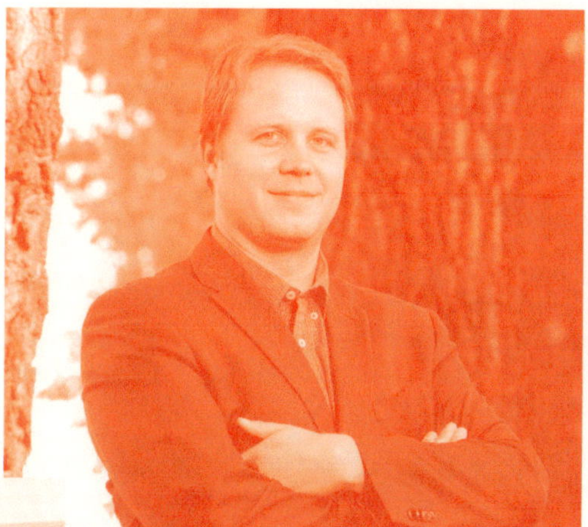

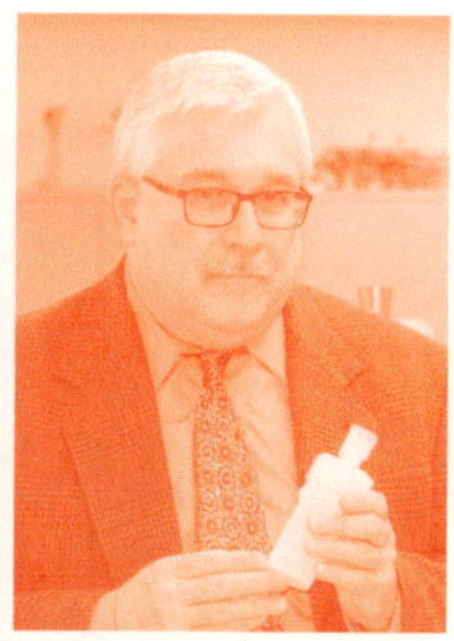

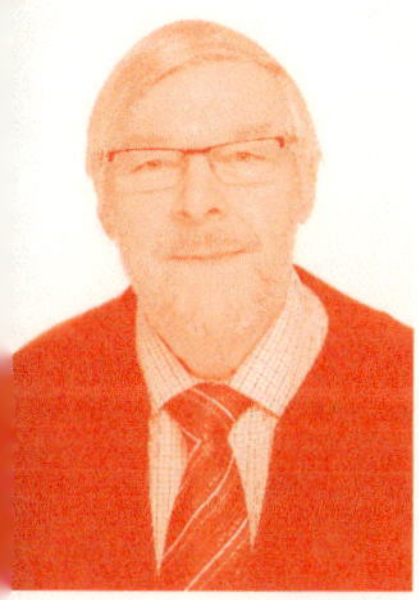

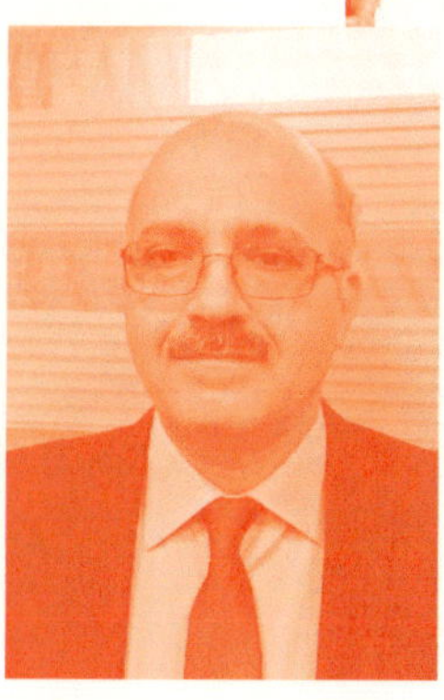

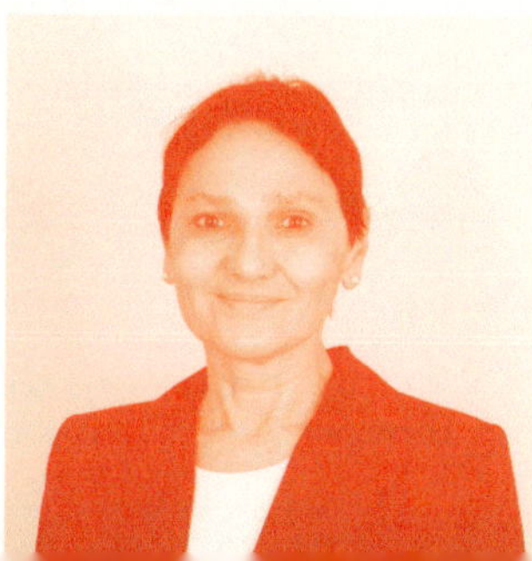

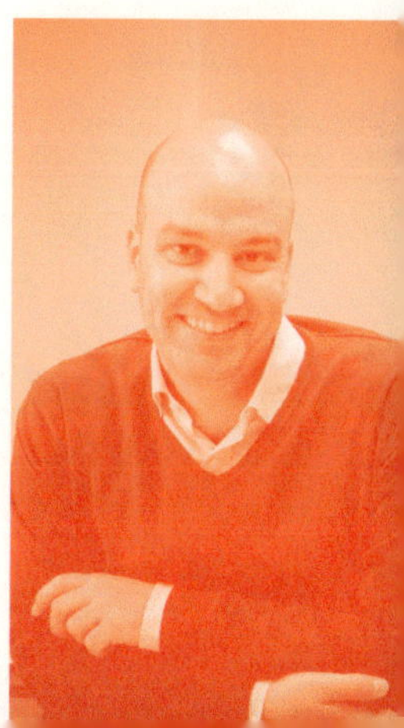

Heavy Metal Toxicity in Public Health
http://dx.doi.org/10.5772/intechopen.83101
Edited by John Kanayochukwu Nduka and Mohamed Nageeb Rashed

Contributors
Paul Seligman, Gamini Siriwardana, Nesrine Boujelben, Marina Alexandrovna Zemlianova, Nina Vladimirovna Zaitseva, Narjala Rama Jyothi, Nainar Abdulkhader Mohamed Farook, Mustafa Ertan Akün, Chanda Siddoo-Atwal, Om Bansal

© The Editor(s) and the Author(s) 2020
The rights of the editor(s) and the author(s) have been asserted in accordance with the Copyright, Designs and Patents Act 1988. All rights to the book as a whole are reserved by INTECHOPEN LIMITED. The book as a whole (compilation) cannot be reproduced, distributed or used for commercial or non-commercial purposes without INTECHOPEN LIMITED's written permission. Enquiries concerning the use of the book should be directed to INTECHOPEN LIMITED rights and permissions department (permissions@intechopen.com).
Violations are liable to prosecution under the governing Copyright Law.

cc BY

Individual chapters of this publication are distributed under the terms of the Creative Commons Attribution 3.0 Unported License which permits commercial use, distribution and reproduction of the individual chapters, provided the original author(s) and source publication are appropriately acknowledged. If so indicated, certain images may not be included under the Creative Commons license. In such cases users will need to obtain permission from the license holder to reproduce the material. More details and guidelines concerning content reuse and adaptation can be found at http://www.intechopen.com/copyright-policy.html.

Notice
Statements and opinions expressed in the chapters are these of the individual contributors and not necessarily those of the editors or publisher. No responsibility is accepted for the accuracy of information contained in the published chapters. The publisher assumes no responsibility for any damage or injury to persons or property arising out of the use of any materials, instructions, methods or ideas contained in the book.

First published in London, United Kingdom, 2020 by IntechOpen
IntechOpen is the global imprint of INTECHOPEN LIMITED, registered in England and Wales, registration number: 11086078, 7th floor, 10 Lower Thames Street, London, EC3R 6AF, United Kingdom
Printed in Croatia

British Library Cataloguing-in-Publication Data
A catalogue record for this book is available from the British Library

Additional hard and PDF copies can be obtained from orders@intechopen.com

Heavy Metal Toxicity in Public Health
Edited by John Kanayochukwu Nduka and Mohamed Nageeb Rashed
p. cm.
Print ISBN 978-1-83880-435-0
Online ISBN 978-1-83880-436-7
eBook (PDF) ISBN 978-1-83880-632-3

For EU product safety concerns:
IN TECH d.o.o., Prolaz Marije Krucifikse Kozulić 3, 51000 Rijeka, Croatia, info@intechopen.com or visit our website at intechopen.com.

We are IntechOpen, the world's leading publisher of Open Access books

Built by scientists, for scientists

4,900+
Open access books available

123,000+
International authors and editors

140M+
Downloads

151
Countries delivered to

Our authors are among the
Top 1%
most cited scientists

12.2%
Contributors from top 500 universities

BOOK CITATION INDEX
CLARIVATE ANALYTICS
INDEXED

WEB OF SCIENCE™

Selection of our books indexed in the Book Citation Index
in Web of Science™ Core Collection (BKCI)

Interested in publishing with us?
Contact book.department@intechopen.com

Numbers displayed above are based on latest data collected.
For more information visit www.intechopen.com

Meet the editors

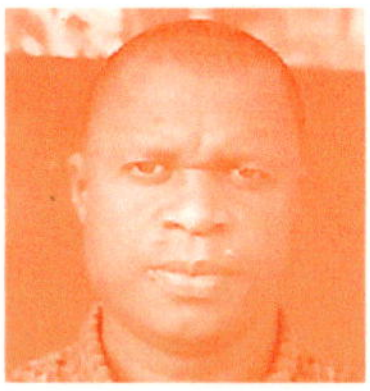

John Kanayochukwu Nduka (PhD) is a member of the Pure and Industrial Chemistry Department of Nnamdi Azikiwe University, Nigeria. He is the head researcher in the Environmental Chemistry and Toxicology Unit and the immediate past head of department. Nduka is one of the most cited authors at Nnamdi Azikiwe University and a number of his papers are indexed in Scopus. He is involved in mentoring young academics at his university and has participated in the National University (NUC) Accreditation of Chemistry Program in a number of Nigerian universities. He received the RULA Award from India for International Best Researcher of 2020 in Environmental Chemistry and Toxicology. He has attended local and international conferences/workshops and delivered public lectures, sizeable numbers of international publications, and has been involved in postgraduate Vivas.

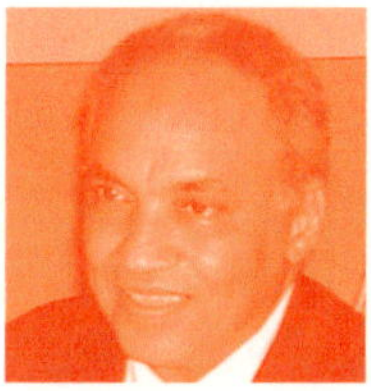

Prof. Mohamed Nageeb Rashed is Professor of Analytical and Environmental Chemistry, and was previously Vice-Dean for Environmental Affairs, Faculty of Science, Aswan University, Egypt. In 1989 he received his PhD in Analytical Environmental Chemistry from Assiut University, Egypt. His research interest is analytical and environmental chemistry with special emphasis on soil and water pollution monitoring, control, and treatment; bioindicators for water pollution monitoring; wastewater impact; advanced oxidation treatment; photocatalysis, nanocatalysts, nanocomposites, and adsorption techniques in water and wastewater treatment. Prof. Rashed has supervised several MSc and PhD theses in the field of pollution and analytical and environmental chemistry. He was selected as an examiner for several PhD theses in analytical chemistry from India, Kazakhstan, and Botswana. Prof. Rashed has published about 90 scientific papers in peer-reviewed international journals. He participated as an invited speaker in 30 international conferences worldwide. Prof. Rashed acts as editor-in-chief and is an editorial board member for several international journals in the fields of chemistry and the environment. His society membership includes several national and international societies. Prof. Rashed was awarded the Egyptian State Award for Environmental Research for the year 2001.

Contents

Preface

Heavy metals have become phenomenal globally. Although extracted from soil/rock as mineral deposits, they are applied industrially in the manufacture of both industrial and consumer goods, reagent chemicals, and engineering materials but are mostly applied in medicine and pharmaceuticals. There is yet no acceptable definition but the greatest problem with heavy metals is environmental contamination, population exposure, and toxicity.

Environmental pollution occurs through the release of heavy metals anthropogenically into water, farmland, and air, and eventually the food web.

Most metals are medically useful but in excess of the healthy limit cause health problems. The increase in non-communicable diseases such as cancer, renal disease, and organ failure may be attributed to exposure to heavy metals.

The chapter "Heavy metal contamination and remediation of water and soil with case studies from Cyprus" examines the heavy metal contamination and remediation of water and soil using a case study. Sewage waters (municipal, agricultural, or industrial) and pesticides are heavy metal laden. Natural resources from the composition of rock formations are the area of study. Heavy metals are found in fruits and vegetables grown on contaminated soil and water and necessitate public health concern globally. Phytoaccumulation, phytostabilization, phytodegradation, phytovolatilization, and hydraulic control methods are also discussed. The author suggested that agricultural soil and water must be carefully investigated before agricultural activities and that acceptable sampling and laboratory analyses should be executed and evaluated accordingly.

The chapter "Sorption of phosphorus, nickel and lead from aqueous solution using manganese oxides coated materials" looks at the rapid development of X-rays in industries such as plating, petrochemicals, and fertilizers, which has led to the discharge of contaminants like phosphorus and heavy metals into the environment. Phosphorus is the key nutrient for the growth of algal and other biological organisms, which cause eutrophication. Methods to eliminate heavy metals from wastewater are chemical precipitation, electrochemical reduction, ion exchange, membrane separation, reverse osmosis, and adsorption. Adsorption involves batch experiments. Both the Freundlich and Langmuir isotherms give a fit to the experimental data for adsorption. To study surface properties of the adsorbents, scanning electron microscopy and X-ray diffraction methods and Brunauer–Emmett–Teller analyses are used. The pseudo-first-order and pseudo-second-order equations as well as the intraparticle diffusion model were determined to test adsorption kinetics and rate constants derived from the three kinetic models being calculated. The pseudo-second-order kinetic model was better appropriated.

The chapter "A role for heavy metal toxicity and air pollution in respiratory tract cancers" reviews cigarette smoke and the health problems it causes: associated lung, nasopharyngeal, and laryngeal cancers, which are connected to its cadmium and lead content. Biomass smoke contents are hazardous, including carbon monoxide, nitrous oxides, sulfur oxides (principally from coal), formaldehyde, and polycyclic organic compounds (notably benzo[a]pyrene). They are implicated in low birth weight, increased infant perinatal mortality, pulmonary tuberculosis, nasopharyngeal and laryngeal cancer, cataracts, and lung cancer, while the harmful effects of free radicals are balanced by the antioxidant action of antioxidant enzymes and non-enzymatic antioxidants that help in the process of detoxification.

The chapter "Mercury toxicity in public health" describes mercury's physical properties, natural and anthropogenic sources, and the differences between liquid and gaseous mercury. Gaseous mercury is poisonous due to the nature of absorption into blood. Mercury 2+ is more poisonous due to high solubility. Exposure and poisoning types are discussed, including Minamata disease.

The chapter "Health risks of potentially toxic metals contaminated water" reviews routes of groundwater and aquatic contamination by toxic metals leaching from toxic industrial waste dumps and municipal landfills, and the leaching of agricultural chemicals from soils. Potentially toxic metals contaminating vegetables, fruits, seafood, and drinking water are the most recognized sources of ingestion by the general public. Toxic metals (Cd, Cu, Pb, Zn, Cr(III), Cr(VI), and Hg) enrich antibiotic-resistant microbes, particularly bacteria by co-selection, because it promotes antibiotic resistance in bacteria even in the absence of antibiotics. Co-selection occurs by co-resistance and cross-resistance.

The chapter "Toxicologic characteristics of nanodisperse manganese oxide" analyzes physical–chemical properties, biological accumulation, and morphological–functional properties at various exposure types. The author experimentally researched nanodisperse MnO_2 water suspension at intragastric, inhalation, and skin-resorptive levels in small rodents (mice and Wistar rats) with various exposure periods. Profound and detailed characteristics of the toxic effects exerted by this substance were found, which determined the target organs and revealed dose-dependent effects. Growth in development and commercialization of nanoindustries and nanotechnological products in the production chain means that such products and technologies are considered to belong to the market segment of new technologies (the sixth technological structure). MnO_2 nanoparticles damage the membranes of astrocytes and neurons and disturb the neurotransmitter ratio. The author detected pathomorphologic brain disorders—hyperemia, subarachnoid hemorrhages, brain edema with perivascular and pericellular spaces dilatation, focuses of nerve fibers, demyelinization, and focal dystrophic changes in vessel endothelium.

The chapter "Intracellular iron concentration and distribution have multiple effects on cell cycle events" reviews how iron depletion causes inhibition of cellular proliferation and cell cycle arrest at different parts of the cell cycle. The chapter explains why in some tissues, particularly rapidly growing cancer cells, iron depletion causes cell cycle arrest and apoptosis, a form of programmed cell death. Other neoplastic tissues are more prone to the toxic effects of iron, which can induce autophagic cell death (termed ferroptosis) via reactive oxygen species resulting in lysosomal degradation of cellular constituents.

The editors John Kanayochukwu Nduka and Mohamed Nageeb Rashed thank the Author Service Manager Ms. Dolores Kuzelj and IntechOpen, UK. The assistance of

Andrea Koric is also noted. We are also grateful to the authors for their hard work and worthy contributions; we have learnt a lot reviewing their chapters. We also thank our families for their understanding.

Editor John Kanayochukwu Nduka is grateful to his wife Ogochukwu and children Chimerem-mma, Onyinye, and Chisom.

John Kanayochukwu Nduka
Environmental Chemistry and Toxicology Research Unit,
Pure and Industrial Chemistry Department,
Nnamdi Azikiwe University,
Awka, Anambra, Nigeria

Mohamed Nageeb Rashed
Department of Chemistry,
Faculty of Science,
Aswan University,
Egypt

Section 1

Environmental Toxic Heavy Metal Pollution and Possible Remediating Techniques

Chapter 1

Heavy Metal Contamination and Remediation of Water and Soil with Case Studies From Cyprus

Mustafa Ertan Akün

Abstract

Some of the heavy metals, (arsenic, cadmium, chromium and nickel) tend to endanger public health, when found above critical limits in soil and water, becoming carcinogenic. The heavy metals are taken by humans through the food chain. As shown by numerous researchers all over the world, the heavy metal contamination mostly come from sewage waters and pesticides, as well as naturally. The natural resources come from the composition of the rock formations present at the area of study. One or all of the above mentioned sources of heavy metal contamination may be present. The study concentrates on the internationally accepted critical limits for soil and water, explains scientific methods of entering into vegetables and fruit, and also tries to shed light on the transfer factors of heavy metals imposing dangers on public health. Remediation of the contaminated soil and water is also discussed, and phytoremediation methods are brought forward, as compared with chemical methods. Details of different phytoremediation (phyto-accumulation, phyto-stabilization, phyto-degradation, phyto-volatilization, and hydraulic control) are also discussed. Actual case studies from North Cyprus are also provided, with real contamination levels observed. Different areas and soil/water/plant species were assessed in detail, displaying concentrations, critical limits, transfer factors, and recommendations.

Keywords: heavy metal, contamination, soil, water, critical limit, public health

1. Introduction

Public health necessitates concentrated efforts of researchers and public authorities and will be under risk if necessary and timely precautions are not undertaken. Soil and groundwaters are inputs for vegetables and fruits and thus animals and mankind as a whole. Sometimes, the sources of heavy metal contamination could as well be airborne. In certain cases, biomonitoring of airborne heavy metal contamination has been an important issue and has been carried out worldwide. Accordingly, during the last few decades, heavy metal contamination of biotic component of environment has attracted the attention of researchers. In this respect, biological materials were used as cheap indicators to determine airborne environmental pollution. Various types of plants (such as lichens, mosses, bark, and leaves of higher plants) were used to detect deposition, accumulation, and distribution of metal pollution and their accumulative potential [1].

IntechOpen

Not only are the heavy metals carcinogenic, but many other diseases such as lung, liver, kidney, and similar diseases are also potential occurrences. Arsenic, cadmium, chromium, and nickel are accepted as group 1 carcinogens by the International Agency for Research on Cancer, and these heavy metals are at the same time utilized commercially [2]. Some other heavy metals are also carcinogenic in nature, and a relevant study listed cobalt, lead, and mercury in addition [3].

Although some of the heavy metals are known to be enhancing the immune system, the same heavy metals above critical limits and some others are hazardous heavy metals for human beings. The critical limits of heavy metals in soil and water are not only different, but they also differ from country to country. Although natural occurrences in different countries and the methods for contamination are the background reasons for this, it is at the same time dependent on the policy makers. Apart from the countries' legislations, some international organizations like the Environmental Protection Agency (EPA) and Food and Agriculture Organization (FAO) also announce and revise these limits periodically. **Table 1** shows critical limits for soils for different countries.

Critical limits of the EPA for water are given below in **Table 2**. The table explains maximum allowable contaminant levels for a wide range of chemicals, either carcinogen or resulting in different health problems.

Numerous researches arrived at scientific findings about the carcinogenic nature of some of the heavy metals and elements. Although not definite and including probability of being a carcinogen, studies reveal the imposed dangers involved, hinting precautions to be taken. Accordingly, the EPA has prepared specific results and cancer descriptors with relevant definitions. **Table 3** below explains cancer descriptors for certain elements.

The heavy metals and carcinogen elements enter the human body via the food chain. The food chain is the mechanism showing the route of heavy metals from soils and waters finally reaching plants, animals, and humans. **Figure 1** shows the journey of heavy metals via food chain.

Thus, public health necessitates to minimize the intake of hazardous heavy metals and elements and if possible to null the amounts. To render this possible, the methodologies by which these metals and elements enter the food chain must be understood correctly, and relevant precautions must be taken.

Country	As	Cd	Cr	Cu	Hg	Ni	Pb	Zn
Australia	20	3	50	100	1	60	300	200
Canada	20	3	250	150	0.8	100	200	500
China	20–40	0.3–0.6	150–300	50–200	0.3–1.0	40–60	80	200–300
Germany	50	5	500	200	5	200	1000	600
Tanzania	1	1	100	200	2	100	200	150
Holland	76	13	180	190	36	100	530	720
NZ	17	3	290	>104	200	N/A	160	N/A
UK	43	1.8	N/A	N/A	26	230	N/A	N/A
USA	0.11	0.48	11	270	1	72	200	1100

Source: [4].

Table 1.
Regulatory standard of heavy metals in agricultural soil (mg/kg).

Chemicals	Maximum contaminant level (mg/L)	Cancer descriptor
Ammonia	—	D
Antimony	0.006	D
Arsenic	010	A
Asbestos	7 MFL	A
Barium	2	N
Beryllium	0.004	—
Boron	—	I
Bromate	0.01	B2
Cadmium	0.005	D
Chloramine3	4^4	—
Chlorine	4^4	D
Chlorine dioxide	0.84	D
Chlorite	1	D
Chromium	0.1	D
Copper	TT^6	D
Cyanide	0.2	I
Fluoride	4	—
Lead	TT^6	B2
Manganese	—	D
Mercury	0.002	D
Molybdenum	—	D
Nickel	—	—
Nitrate	10	—
Nitrite	1	—
Nitrate + Nitrite	10	—
Perchlorate2	—	L/N
Selenium	0.05	D
Silver	—	D
Strontium	—	D
Thallium	0.002	I
White phosphorous	—	D
Zinc	—	

Source: [5].

Table 2.
Standards of heavy metals in water and health advisories.

Descriptor	Definition
A	Human carcinogen
B	Probable human carcinogen
B1	Indicates limited human evidence
B2	Indicates sufficient evidence in animals and inadequate or no evidence in humans
C	Possible human carcinogen

Descriptor	Definition
D	Not classifiable as to human carcinogenicity
E	Evidence of non-carcinogenicity for humans
H	Carcinogenic to humans
I	Inadequate information to assess carcinogenic potential
L	Likely to be carcinogenic to humans
N	Not likely to be carcinogenic to humans
L/N	Likely to be carcinogenic above a specified dose but not likely to be carcinogenic below that dose because a key event in tumor formation does not occur below that dose
S	Suggestive evidence of carcinogenic potential

Source: [5].

Table 3.
Cancer descriptors.

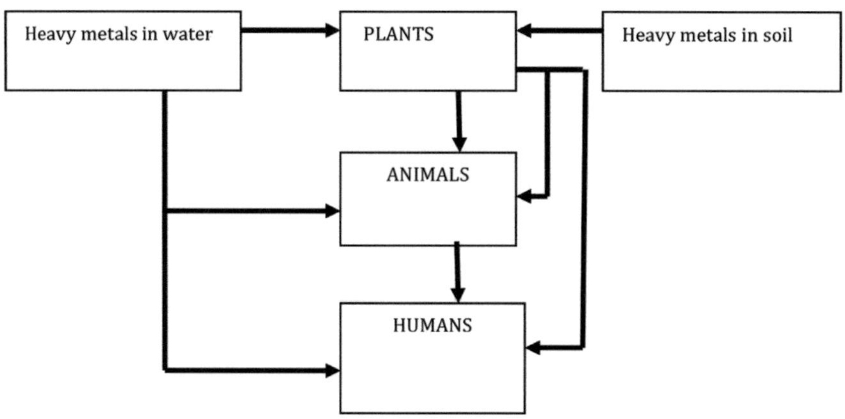

Figure 1.
Journey of heavy metals via food chain.

2. Soil and water contamination and remediation/precautions

There are numerous sources of heavy metal contamination of soils and water. These are briefly explained below:

a. ***Sewage waters***: This is an anthropogenic activity. The sewage waters are those collected via municipal, agricultural, and industrial origin [6]. The potential heavy metal inclusions from these sources are normally collected at treatment plants. Treatment results are never theoretically 100% efficient, and following the treatment process, disposed water is mostly utilized in irrigation of agricultural areas. The irrigation process then transfers the heavy metal content to soils and groundwaters.

b. ***Pesticides***: This is an anthropogenic activity. Many plants (vegetables, fruits, and trees) are under the attack of certain pests and are not only decreasing the quality of the products but also contaminating them with heavy metals, due to the presence of such. The research carried out on the heavy metal levels of spinach [7] following the application of pesticides (DELVAP 1000 EC) displayed that the concentrations before and after the pesticide application changed significantly. The application of pesticides also contaminates the soil in the surrounding, and the included heavy metals may also reach the groundwaters.

c. ***Natural resources***: This is a natural activity. Many elements and heavy metals can be naturally present in the surrounding, and erosion of these rock formations including such elements and heavy metals can be transformed into soil. Downward percolation of rain waters may as well result in the arrival of such to groundwaters. A related research forwards that under different and certain environmental conditions, natural emissions of heavy metals occur that may in turn lead to the release of metals from their endemic spheres to different environment compartments [8].

2.1 Types of remediation

The remediation methodologies can be chemical or biological in nature. Since heavy metal contamination itself is a chemical process, chemical remediation should be avoided, and biological processes should be introduced. The phytoremediation of heavy metals from the contaminated sites generally happens through any one or more of the following mechanisms or processes [9]: "phyto-accumulation," "phyto-stabilization," "phyto-degradation," "phyto-volatilization," and "hydraulic control."

2.1.1 Phyto-accumulation

Phyto-accumulation is a mechanism through which heavy metals in soil and water at a specific region are accumulated in native plants and are disposed thereafter. In a research carried out in Pakistan [10], heavy metal accumulation in crops and soils from wastewater irrigation was realized via the usage of *Cannabis sativa* L., *Chenopodium album* L., *Datura stramonium* L., *Sonchus asper* L., *Amaranthus viridis* L., *Oenothera rosea* (LHer), *Xanthium stramonium* L., Polygonum macalosa L., *Nasturtium officinale* L., and *Conyza canadensis* L. Metal concentrations are in the order iron (Fe) > zinc (Zn) > chromium (Cr) > nickel (Ni) > cadmium (Cd). Most of the species accumulated more heavy metals in roots than shoots. Among species, the concentrations were in the order *C. sativa* > *C. album* > *X. stramonium* > *C. canadensis* > *A. viridis* > *N. officinale* > *P. macalosa* > *D. stramonium* > *S. asper* > *O. rosea*.

In this mechanism, bio-concentration factor (BCF) and biological absorption coefficient (BAC) are also important parameters to be considered. According to the international guidelines, "bioaccumulation" is the process where chemical concentration in an aquatic organism reaches a level that exceeds that in the water as a result of chemical uptake through all routes of chemical exposure. Bioaccumulation takes place under field conditions and is a combination of chemical bio-concentration and biomagnification.

On the other hand, metal accumulation is expressed by the metal biological absorption coefficient (BAC) or the plant-to-soil/water metal concentration ratio. Bio-concentration factors are used to relate pollutant residues in aquatic organisms to the pollutant concentration in ambient waters. Many chemical compounds, especially those with a hydrophobic component, partition easily into the lipids and lipid membranes of organisms and bioaccumulate.

BCF and BAC are described by the following formulas:

$$BCF = CB/CWD = k1/(k2 + kE + kM + kG) \quad (1)$$

$$BAC = CB/CWD = \{k1 + kD\ (CB/CWD)\}/(k2 + kE + kM + kG) \quad (2)$$

where CB is the chemical concentration in the organism (g/kg^{-1}), k1 is the chemical uptake rate constant from the water at the respiratory surface ($L{\cdot}kg^{-1}{\cdot}d^{-1}$), CWD is the freely dissolved chemical concentration in the water ($g{\cdot}L^{-1}$), kD is the uptake rate constant for chemical in the diet ($kg \times kg^{-1} \times d^{-1}$), and k2, kE, kM, and kG are rate constants (d^{-1}) representing chemical elimination from the organism via the respiratory surface, fecal egestion, metabolic biotransformation, and growth dilution, respectively.

Phyto-accumulation for arsenic was adopted in India and Bangladesh by utilizing two different plant species, namely, *Pteris vittata* and *Chrysopogon zizanioides*. Laboratory scale studies gave way to observations regarding growth of these plants in different concentrations of 10–50 mg As/kg soil. Arsenic accumulation in leaves, stem, and root were analyzed at different time intervals, observing survival of plants. Results were encouraging, and it was observed that they could accumulate significant amounts of arsenic [11].

2.1.2 Phyto-stabilization

Phyto-stabilization comprises the establishment of a plant cover on the surface of the contaminated sites for reducing the mobility of contaminants within the vadose zone via accumulation by roots or immobilization within the rhizosphere, reducing off-site contamination [12]. The process includes transpiration and root growth that immobilizes contaminants by reducing leaching, controlling erosion, creating an aerobic environment in the root zone, and adding organic matter to the substrate that binds the contaminant.

Microbial activity related with the plant roots may accelerate the degradation of organic contaminants such as pesticides and hydrocarbons to nontoxic forms. Phyto-stabilization can be enhanced by using soil amendments that immobilize metal(loid)s combined with plant species that are tolerant of high levels of contaminants and low-fertility soils or tailings. Although effective in the containment of metal(loid)s, the site requires regular monitoring to ensure that the stabilizing conditions are maintained. Soil amendments used to enhance immobilization may need to be periodically reapplied to maintain their effectiveness.

2.1.3 Phyto-degradation

Phyto-degradation, which is also known as phyto-transformation, is the breakdown of contaminants taken up by plants through metabolic processes within the plant or the breakdown of contaminants surrounding the plant through the effect of enzymes produced by the plants. Plants are able to produce enzymes that catalyze and accelerate degradation. Hence, organic pollutants are broken down into simpler molecular forms and are incorporated into plant tissues to aid plant growth.

Figure 2 shows the degradation process. Enzymes in plant roots break down (degrade) organic contaminants. The fragments are incorporated into new plant material.

A relevant research [13] put forth that the phyto-degradation of organic compounds can take place inside the plant or within the rhizosphere of the plant.

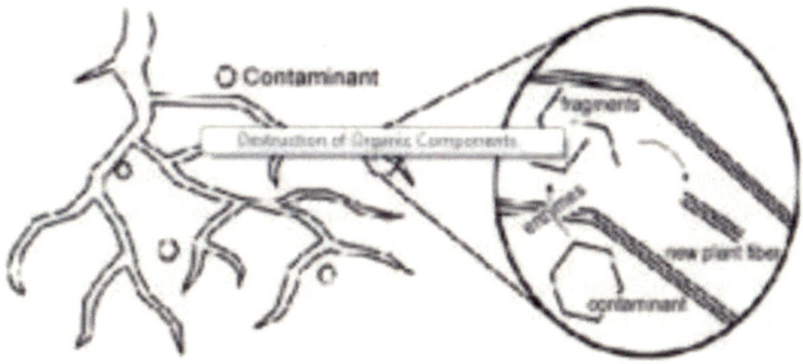

Figure 2.
Degradation process.

Many different compounds and compound classes can be removed from the environment by phyto-degradation, including solvents in groundwater, petroleum and aromatic compounds in soils, and volatile compounds in the air. Although currently a relatively new area of research, studies regarding the underlying science necessary for a wide range of applications for plant-based remediation of organic contaminants are continuing.

2.1.4 Phyto-volatilization

Phyto-volatilization is a process where plants take up contaminants from soil and release them as volatile form into the atmosphere via transpiration. The process occurs as growing plants absorb water and organic contaminants.

It is possible for plants to interact with a variety of organic compounds and affect the fate and transport of many environmental contaminants. Volatile organic compounds may be volatilized from stems or leaves (direct phyto-volatilization) or from soil due to plant root activities (indirect phyto-volatilization) [14]. Fluxes of contaminants volatilizing from plants range from local contaminant spills to global fluxes of methane emanating biochemically reducing organic carbon. In this article past studies are reviewed to differentiate between direct and indirect phyto-volatilization. Findings of the study revealed that compounds with low octanol-air partitioning coefficients are more likely to be phyto-volatilized. Reports of direct phyto-volatilization compared favorably to model predictions. **Figure 3** represents direct and indirect phyto-volatilization.

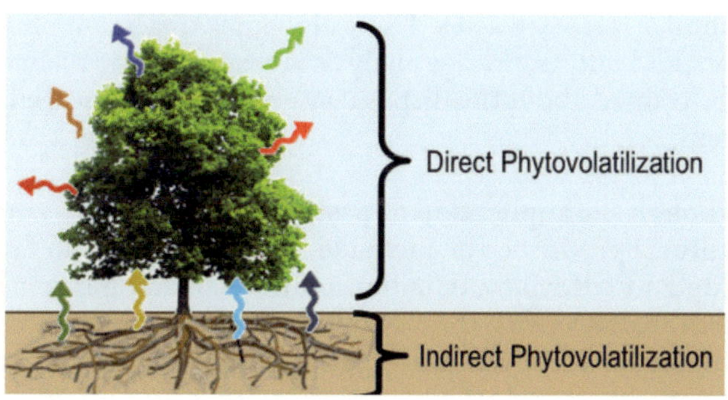

Figure 3.
Direct and indirect phyto-volatilization.

2.1.5 Hydraulic control

Hydraulic control is the method of phytoremediation, where the contaminated aqueous medium's flow direction is altered and contaminated flow is oriented. The relevant research study [15] designed such a system at the field.

The goal of this hydraulic capture model for remediation purposes was to design a well field so that the groundwater flow direction was altered. In so doing, halting or reversing the migration of a contaminant plume was made possible. Management strategies typically require a well design that will contain or shrink a plume at minimum cost. Objective functions and constraints can be nonlinear, non-convex, non-differentiable, or even discontinuous. Computational efficiency and accuracy is normally desirable and often affects the solution method.

2.2 Precautions against soil and water contamination

The precautions against contamination also differ according to the sources of contamination.

Accordingly, the precautions according to the sources are provided below:

a. ***Sewage waters***: The *municipal* sewage waters are those connected from houses at inhabited areas. Hazardous elements and heavy metals may enter the system from any location by any liquid or solid. The inhabitants must be trained about the disposal system at the start point to minimize their entrance into the system. Frequent analysis of input and output at the treatment plant must be carried out; methods of minimizing contamination levels must be employed; and output containing hazardous elements and heavy metals with lower than critical limits must be used for irrigation purposes. The *agricultural* sewage waters are those collected at the farms and greenhouses used for cleaning purposes. These may from time to time include disposed plant parts, some soil, and some fertilizers. Thus, probability of presence of hazardous elements and heavy metals is quite high, and serious precautions are necessary. These are also entering the treatment plants, and like municipal sewage waters, the relevant people must again be trained about the disposal system at the start point to minimize their entrance into the system. Frequent analysis of input and output at the treatment plant must again be carried out; methods of minimizing contamination levels must be employed; and output containing hazardous elements and heavy metals with lower than critical limits must be used for irrigation purposes. The most dangerous of the types of sewage waters is definitely *industrial* sewage waters. This group includes slaughterhouse waste, whey of milk processing factories, paint factory waste, animal breeding waste, and similar factory wastes. These also enter treatment plants, and again frequent input and output sewage analysis is required. The relevant people must again be trained about the disposal system to minimize their entrance into the system.

b. ***Pesticides***: Though the application of pesticides is connected with the quality of the agricultural products, the included heavy metals are in fact decreasing the quality and reliability. In many countries, many pesticide types are banned in conformance with the technological advancements and information regarding heavy metals. A study carried out in Nigeria showed the presence of heavy metals (Pb, As, Cd, Cr, and Zn) in different parts of the plants and at different concentrations, with some above the WHO/FAO permissible limits [16]. At some instances, it may become must to apply the pesticide, and under such circumstances, the adequate dose must be applied by expert personnel.

c. ***Natural resources***: Just like the areas polluted by anthropogenic activities, in case of natural occurrence of heavy metals also, bioremediation can be an effective precaution. A relevant research titled "**Heavy Metal Polluted Soils: Effect on Plants and Bioremediation Methods**" in 2014 applied bioremediation and analyzed the results [17]. Microorganisms and plants employ different mechanisms for the bioremediation of polluted soils. Using plants for the treatment of polluted soils is a more common approach in the bioremediation of heavy metal polluted soils. Combining both microorganisms and plants is an approach to bioremediation that ensures a more efficient cleanup of heavy metal polluted soils. However, success of this approach largely depends on the species of organisms involved in the process.

3. Case studies of soil and water contamination from Cyprus

3.1 Arsenic, cadmium, and lead distribution of Cyprus soils

Selected locations in Cyprus were investigated by the Cancer Research Fund and Frederick Institute of Technology in search of distribution of heavy metals. The collaborative research investigated for lead, arsenic, and cadmium [18]. The observations of cancer incidents triggered the research all over the island, and the findings displayed contamination at certain areas. To achieve an analytical distribution, 260 composite soil samples (140 from North Cyprus and 120 from South Cyprus) were investigated for the presence of heavy metal contamination. The soil samples were obtained from Güzelyurt Bostancı, Yuvacık, Lefkoşa, Karpaz, Alevkayası, Kırnı, and Mesarya in North Cyprus. The concentration of lead in these areas ranged between 8 and 45 ppm, while that of arsenic ranged between 8 and 15 ppm and that of cadmium ranged between 0 and 0.7 ppm. These findings are given in **Table 4**.

In South Cyprus, the soil samples were obtained from Dali, Sotira, Omodos, Acheleia, Polis, and Evrychou. The concentration of lead in these areas ranged between 6 and 53 ppm, while that of arsenic ranged between 6 and 19 ppm and that of cadmium ranged between 0 and 0.4 ppm, given below in **Table 5**.

Area	Pb (ppm)	As (ppm)	Cd (ppm)
Alevkayası	32.58	11.25	0.34
Lefkoşa	44.29	11.87	0.69
Kırnı	40.51	14.63	0.47
Yuvacık	32.42	8.98	0.34
Bostancı	8.02	9.47	0.2
Mesarya	12.6	11.09	0.33
Karpaz	17.19	13.56	0.3
Source: [18]			

Table 4.
Distribution of lead, arsenic, and cadmium in North Cyprus.

Area	Pb (ppm)	As (ppm)	Cd (ppm)
Dali	10.25	7.17	0.39
Sotira	14.02	11.68	0.26
Omodos	6.81	6.37	0.20
Acheleia	20.58	10.06	0.35
Evrychou	52.39	18.30	0.26
Polis	13.59	12.43	0.23

Source: [18]

Table 5.
Distribution of lead, arsenic, and cadmium in South Cyprus.

The regulatory standards given in **Table 1** hints that lead can be at safe concentrations but arsenic and cadmium need attention and may be regarded as present at above critical limits.

3.2 Heavy metal contamination of agricultural soils of Yedidalga abandoned copper mine

At Yedidalga harbor of abandoned copper mine at North Cyprus, agricultural soils were investigated for levels of soil contamination by heavy metals. **Figure 4** shows the study area and the sampling locations.

Copper, lead, chromium, cadmium, and zinc concentrations were investigated on samples collected at nine different locations. The heavy metal contents were

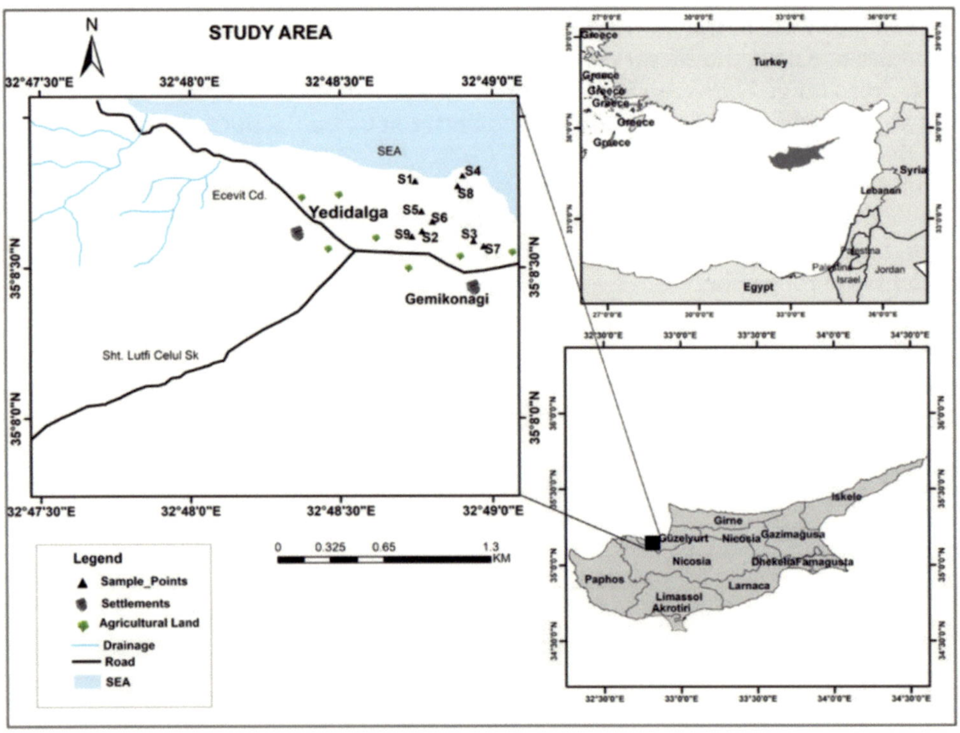

Figure 4.
Study area and sampling locations [19].

determined using atomic absorption spectrophotometer (AAS). The results obtained are presented in **Figure 5**.

The findings displayed average concentration levels (mg/kg) as follows: Cu, 208.4; Pb, 119.4; Cr, 18.38; Cd, 6.19; and Zn, 144.2. The corresponding critical limits of the same heavy metals are as follows: Cu, 13–24; Pb, 22–44; Cr, 12–83; Cd, 0.37–0.78; and Zn, 45–100. Accordingly, there is significant pollution of Cu, Pb, Cd, and Zn, while there is no pollution with respect to Cr.

The study also evaluated the level of contamination and assessed the potential ecological risk posed by heavy metals. Several quantitative indices were utilized to assess the soil pollution status. Results revealed that comparatively all heavy metals exceeded the background values. The peak values were observed in the soils from the locations close to the Yedidalga farming lands. Spatial distribution of pollution load index (PLI) and potential ecological risk index (RI) is given in **Figure 6**.

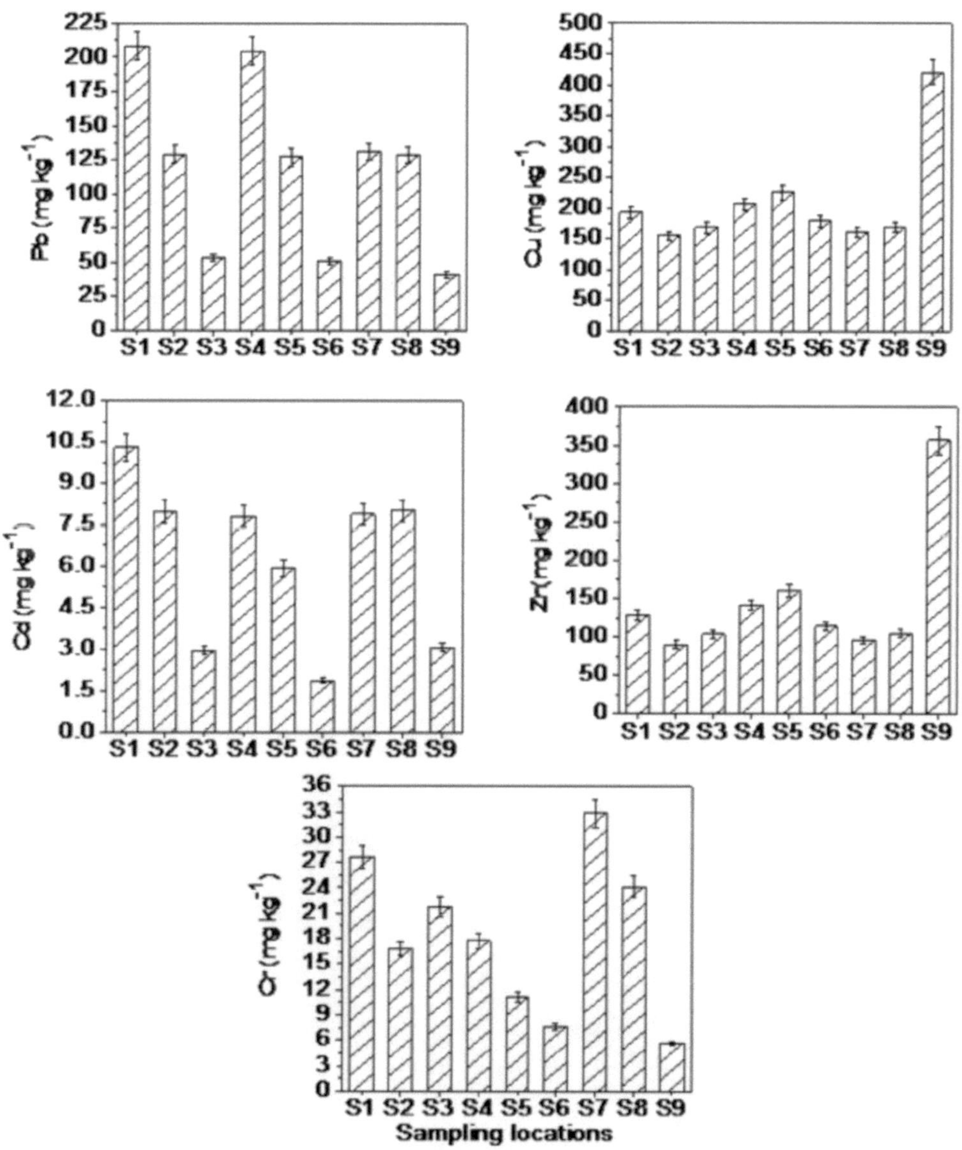

Figure 5.
Heavy metal contamination levels at Yedidalga harbor [19].

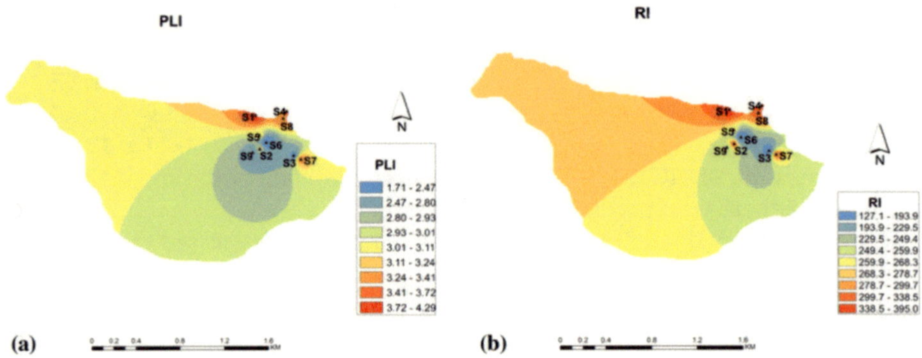

Figure 6.
Spatial distributions of PLI and RI [19].

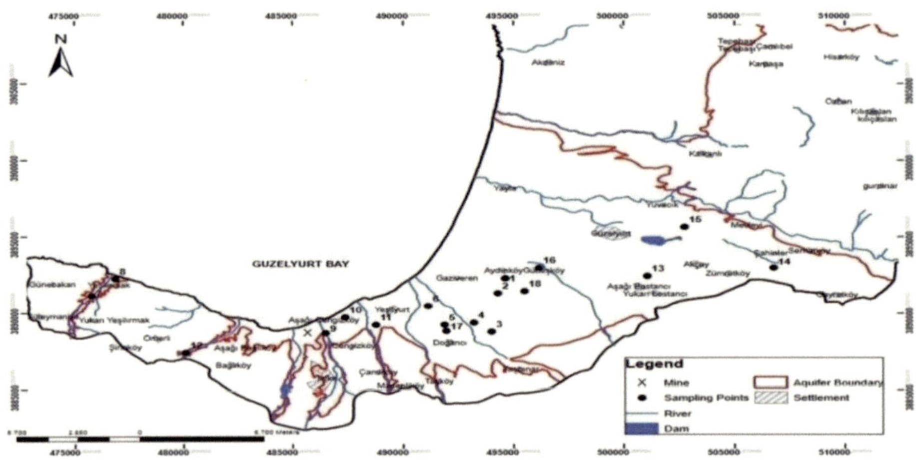

Figure 7.
Sample collecting locations [20].

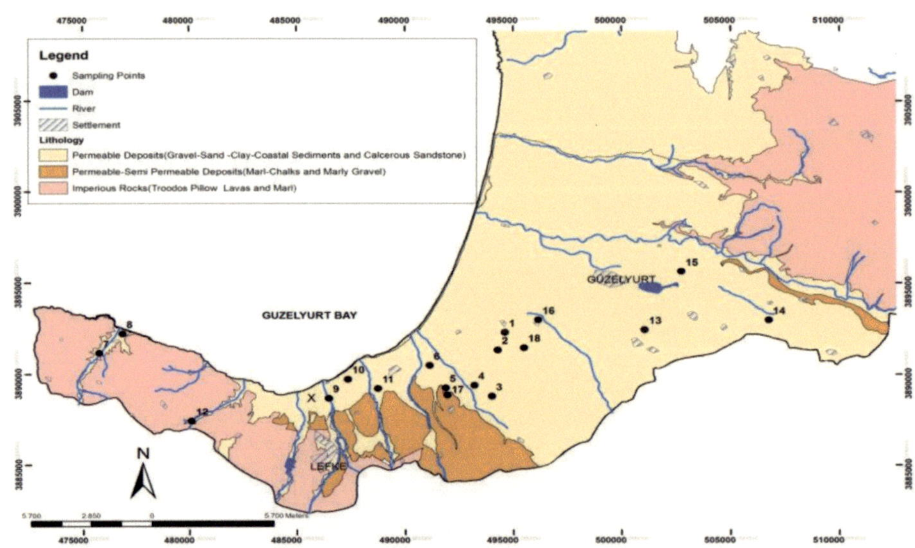

Figure 8.
Geological nature of study area [20].

Sample no	As (μg/L)	Cd (μg/L)	Cr (μg/L)	Hg (μg/L)	Pb (μg/L)	Fe (μg/L)
1	2.95 ± 0.02	<0.01	6.97 ± 0.19	0.11 ± 0.006	<0.01	1266.9 ± 11.55
2	0.71 ± 0.03	<0.01	12.16 ± 0.06	0.03 ± 0.01	0.24 ± 0.01	305.24 ± 0.88
3	0.47 ± 0.03	<0.01	5.79 ± 0.06	0.03 ± 0.01	1.09 ± 0.01	310.57 ± 4.26
4	0.41 ± 0.00	<0.01	5.78 ± 0.18	0.01 ± 0.01	1.25 ± 0.03	260.57 ± 9.67
5	0.93 ± 0.04	<0.01	14.46 ± 0.10	0.02 ± 0.01	<0.01	186.57 ± 6.84
6	1.43 ± 0.05	<0.01	8.10 ± 0.03	0.03 ± 0.01	1.40 ± 0.05	392.24 ± 1.76
7	0.05 ± 0.01	0.02 ± 0.01	0.32 ± 0.01	<0.01	0.21 ± 0.01	294.90 ± 14.64
8	0.61 ± 0.02	0.03 ± 0.01	0.57 ± 0.01	0.01 ± 0.01	<0.01	602.24 ± 3.48
9	0.19 ± 0.01	0.03 ± 0.01	0.85 ± 0.01	<0.01	0.01 ± 0.003	600.90 ± 25.48
10	1.12 ± 0.01	0.04 ± 0.01	7.44 ± 0.08	0.03 ± 0.01	<0.01	686.90 ± 1.53
11	0.18 ± 0.01	0.01 ± 0.01	9.31 ± 0.12	0.01 ± 0.01	0.03 ± 0.01	313.90 ± 2.89
12	0.12 ± 0.01	0.01 ± 0.01	0.13 ± 0.01	<0.01	0.26 ± 0.01	532.90 ± 7.55
13	0.92 ± 0.01	0.08 ± 0.01	9.55 ± 0.30	<0.01	0.71 ± 0.02	2253.57 ± 61.73
14	0.32 ± 0.03	0.01 ± 0.01	1.17 ± 0.09	<0.01	0.63 ± 0.01	302.90 ± 4.16
15	0.88 ± 0.01	0.03 ± 0.01	2.25 ± 0.02	0.01 ± 0.01	2.79 ± 0.03	370.24 ± 3.76
16	1.49 ± 0.02	<0.01	12.42 ± 0.07	0.02 ± 0.01	0.33 ± 0.03	577.90 ± 0.58
17	0.63 ± 0.01	0.01 ± 0.01	13.39 ± 0.17	0.01 ± 0.01	0.67 ± 0.02	386.90 ± 6.08
18	3.07 ± 0.02	<0.01	11.86 ± 0.01	0.03 ± 0.01	0.68 ± 0.01	754.24 ± 3.84

Table 6.
Heavy metal distribution of Güzelyurt agricultural waters.

Pollution load index graded the overall studied area as moderately–heavily contaminated level. Potential ecological risk analysis forwarded that the ecological risk level indicated that 55.6% of sampling locations exceeded 300 (RI > 300). These study results definitely suggest that pollution precautions must be implemented. The main cause of accumulation of these metals is found to be related with the presence of mine wastes at Yedidalga mine harbor.

3.3 Quality and heavy metal contamination of Güzelyurt agricultural waters

The most active agricultural region of Güzelyurt in North Cyprus was investigated with respect to agricultural quality and heavy metal content. At the same time, the aim of the research is to shed light on the irrigation water management in the said region and to assess the groundwater quality. The management methodology was studied, and representative groundwater samples collected from different villages (**Figure 7**) were analyzed for physicochemical parameters and contamination [20].

Within the scope of the study, the geological nature of the study area is also effective and is given in **Figure 8**.

The research put forth that the concentration of heavy metals was all below the FAO guideline threshold limits, following the order Fe > Cr > As>Pb > Hg > Cd. **Table 6** displays the distribution of heavy metals at the study area.

Main cations, on the other hand, indicated $Na^+ > Mg^{2+} > Ca^{2+} > K^+$, while that of anions displayed $Cl^- > HCO_3^- > SO_4^{2-} > CO_3^{2-}$ that comply with irrigation water standards. Seawater intrusion was determined by Revelle index; piper diagram indicated Ca^{2+}-Mg^{2+}-Cl^- as the major hydro chemical facies; and USSL salinity diagram was also used for salinity and sodium hazard. Irrigation water quality was evaluated by sodium adsorption ratio (SAR), residual sodium carbonate, percent of sodium, magnesium adsorption ratio (MAR), Kelly's index, total hardness, permeability index, residual Mg^{2+}/Ca^{2+} ratio, and electrical conductivity. Only SAR values displayed perfect groundwater quality, while others showed good quality, except for MAR, which was unsuitable.

In conclusion, the study put forth in general the safe use of the groundwater for the purpose of irrigation. High amounts of Mg^{2+} in water resulted in unsuitable MAR values. Majority of groundwater samples were in the field of Ca^{2+}-Mg^{2+}-Cl^- water types. Lack of water management policies brings problems to farmers.

4. Conclusion

Heavy metal contamination of water and soil is dangerous to human life; but the issue becomes much critical when the region in question is an agricultural region. The reason behind this is the entrance of natural or anthropogenic potential hazardous heavy metals into the human body via food chain. Not only conventional diseases but various cancer diseases are also observed as a result of research studies.

Consequently, agricultural soil and water must be carefully investigated before the initiation of the agricultural activities. Acceptable sampling and laboratory analyses should be executed and evaluated accordingly. In this respect, sources of contamination (natural or anthropogenic) have to be identified and analyzed for the presence of contamination.

In case of presence of contamination of soil and water by heavy metals, and if the concentrations are above the acceptable limits, necessary and timely precautions must be taken. Of the general biological and chemical methods of remediation, the former should be preferred, so as not to introduce new chemicals to the medium.

The method of remediation must be selected among *phyto-accumulation*, *phyto-stabilization*, *phyto-degradation*, *phyto-volatilization*, and *hydraulic control*. There are numerous researches which discuss different types of plant species getting rid of heavy metals through different methods, without introducing new chemical contaminations.

Such research should not only be left on paper and must be implemented in agricultural regions all over the world, with the objective of enhancing the health and well-being of the humans. Creating necessary awareness in areas of potential contamination through social responsibility projects will enhance such studies.

Author details

Mustafa Ertan Akün
Faculty of Engineering, Cancer Research Foundation, Biotechnology Research Center, Environmental Research Center, Cyprus International University, Turkish Republic of North Cyprus, Turkey

*Address all correspondence to: eakun@ciu.edu.tr

IntechOpen

© 2020 The Author(s). Licensee IntechOpen. This chapter is distributed under the terms of the Creative Commons Attribution License (http://creativecommons.org/licenses/by/3.0), which permits unrestricted use, distribution, and reproduction in any medium, provided the original work is properly cited.

References

[1] Mehran H, Mitra A, Payam N. Bio-monitoring of airborne heavy metal contamination. In: Air Pollution: Monitoring, Modelling, Health and Control. IntechOpen, London-UK; Vol. 20. 2012. DOI: 10.5772/32963

[2] Hyun K, Yeo JK, Young RS. An overview of carcinogenic heavy metal: Molecular toxicity mechanism and prevention. Journal of Cancer Prevention. 2015;**20**(4):232. DOI: 10.15430/JCP.2015.20.4.232

[3] Preeyaporn K, Young RS. Advances in carcinogenic metal toxicity and potential molecular markers. International Journal of Molecular Sciences. 2011;**12**:9576-9595. DOI: 10.3390/ijms12129576

[4] Bakshi S, Banik C, He Z. The impact of heavy metal contamination on soil health. In: Managing Soil Health for Sustainable Agriculture. Burleigh Dodds Series In Agricultural Science, USA Vol. 2. 2018. pp. 63-95. DOI: 10.19103/AS.2017.0033.20

[5] Environmental Pollution Agency, EPA. Edition of the Drinking Water Standards and Health Advisories Tables; 2018

[6] Behbahaninia A, Mirbagheri SA, Khorasani N, Nouri J, Javid AH. Heavy metal contamination of municipal effluent in soil and plants. Journal of Food, Agriculture and Environment. 2009;**7**(3-4):851-856

[7] Chiroma TM, Abdulkarim BI, Kefas HM. The impact of pesticide application on heavy metal (Cd, Pb and Cu) levels in spinach. Leonardo Electronic Journal of Practices and Technologies. 2007;**11**:117-122. Available from: https://www.researchgate.net/publication/26492971

[8] Masindi V, Muedi KL. Environmental contamination by heavy metals. In: Heavy Metals. Rijeka: Intech Open; 2018. pp. 115-133. DOI: 10.5772/intechopen.76082

[9] Muthusaravanan S, Sivarajasekar N, Vivek JS, Paramasivan T, Naushad M, Prakashmaran J, et al. Phytoremediation of heavy metals: Mechanisms, methods and enhancements. Environmental Chemistry Letters. 2018;**16**(4):1339-1359. DOI: 10.1007/s10311-018-0762-3

[10] Irshad M, Ruqia B, Hussain Z. Heavy phytoaccumulation of heavy metals in natural vegetation at the municipal wastewater site in Abbottabad, Pakistan. International Journal of Phytoremediation. 2015;**17**(12):1269-1273. DOI: 10.1080/15226514.2014.950409

[11] Sateesh NH. Removal of arsenic by phyto-re mediation- a study of two plant species. International Journal of Scientific Engineering and Technology. 2012;**1**(5):218-224

[12] Bolan NS, Park JH, Robinson B, Naidu R, Huh KY. Phytostabilization: A green approach to contaminant containment. Advances in Agronomy. 2011;**112**:145-204. DOI: 10.1016/B978-0-12-385538-1.00004-4

[13] Newman LA, Reynolds CM. Phyto-degradation of organic compounds. Current Opinion in Biotechnology. 2004;**15**(3):225-230. DOI: 10.1016/j.copbio.2004.04.006

[14] Limmer M, Burken J. Phyto-Volatilization of Organic Contaminants. USA: American Chemical Society; 2016. DOI: 10.1021/acs.est.5b04113

[15] Fowler KR, Kelley CT, Kees CE, Miller CT. A hydraulic capture application for optimal remediation design. Developments in Water Science. 2004;**55**(Part 2):1149-1157. DOI: 10.1016/S0167-5648(04)80131-X

[16] Barau BW, Abdulhameed A, Ezra AG, Muhammad M, Kyari EM, Bawa U. Heavy metal contamination of some vegetables from pesticides and the potential health risk in Bauchi, northern Nigeria. Affrev Stech: An International Journal of Science and Technology. 2018;7(1):1-11. DOI: 10.4314/stech.v7i1.1

[17] Chibuike GU, Obiora SC. Heavy Metal Polluted Soils: Effect on Plants and Bioremediation Methods. Vol. 2014. UK: Hindawi Publishing Corporation, Applied and Environmental Soil Science; 2014. p. 752708. 1-12. DOI: 10.1155/2014/752708

[18] Akun ME, Yamacı RF, Charalambous C, Lechtvich S, Djamgoz MBA. The distribution of carcinogenic heavy metals in Cyprus soil. In: Conversion of Agricultural Wastes into Value Added Product with high Protein Content by Growing *Pleurotus ostreatus*. Switzerland Springer; 2011. pp. 353-359. DOI: 10.1007/978-3-540-95991-5_33

[19] Barkett MO, Akün E. Heavy metal contents of contaminated soils and ecological risk assessment in abandoned copper mine harbor in Yedidalga, Northern Cyprus. Environment and Earth Science. 2019;77:378. DOI: 10.1007/s12665-018-7556-6

[20] Arslan B, Akün E. Management, contamination and quality evaluation of groundwater in North Cyprus. Agricultural Water Management. 2019;**222**:1-11. DOI: 10.1016/j.agwat.2019.05.023

Chapter 2

Sorption of Phosphorus, Nickel, and Lead from Aqueous Solution Using Manganese Oxide-Coated Materials

Nesrine Boujelben

Abstract

Manganese oxide-coated sand (MOCS) and manganese oxide-coated crushed brick (MOCB) were prepared and characterized and employed for the removal of phosphorus ions (PO_4^{3-}) and Pb(II) and Ni(II) ions from aqueous solution. To study the surface properties of the adsorbents, scanning electron microscopy (SEM), X-ray diffraction (XRD) methods, and BET analyses were used. Adsorption was investigated by batch experiments. The estimated optimum pH was 7 for Ni(II) and 5 for all other ions retention by the two considered adsorbents. Both the Freundlich and Langmuir isotherms provided a reasonable fit to the experimental data for the adsorption. The adsorption capacities of the coated adsorbents at a considered pH value and a temperature of 20°C were 1.96 and 2.08 mg/g for PO_4^{3-}, 2.4 and 3.33 mg/g for Ni(II), and 6 and 6.25 for Pb(II) onto MOCS and MOCB, respectively. The pseudo-first-order and pseudo-second-order equations as well as the intraparticle diffusion model were determined to test the adsorption kinetics and the rate constants derived from the three kinetic models being calculated. The pseudo-second-order kinetic model was better appropriated. Results obtained from this study confirm that the manganese oxide-coated sorbent is considerably considered like suitable for the removal of anions and cations from aqueous solutions.

Keywords: manganese oxide-coated sorbents, nickel copper and lead removal, phosphorus ions, kinetic study, thermodynamic parameters

1. Introduction

Due to the rapid development of such industries as plating, petrochemicals, and fertilizers, there has been excessive discharge of contaminant, like phosphorus and heavy metals, into the environment, resulting in health hazards [1]. Phosphorus is the key nutrient for the growth of algal and other biological organisms, which in excess causes eutrophication of water bodies and heavy metals such as lead and nickel, which are harmful and can cause disease and damage to human health if present above certain concentrations [2, 3]. For this reason, it is important to remove them from wastewater before it is discharged into the environment [2]. There are many methods to eliminate heavy metals from wastewater [2], including chemical precipitation [4], electrochemical reduction [5], ion exchange [6],

 IntechOpen

membrane separation, reverse osmosis [7], and adsorption [8–10]. Adsorption is considered the most effective one due to its properties of simple operation, low cost, and high efficiency over a wide concentration range of pollutants [11]. Typical adsorbents which have been extensively employed to remove heavy metals are clay minerals [12], carbon-based materials [13], and metal oxides [14]. Recently, different types of low-cost natural and modified minerals for the removal of heavy metals from aqueous solutions have been used. Due to the high surface charge density, various Mn oxides (e.g., including pyrolusite (β-MnO_2) and birnessite (σ-MnO_2)) have been extensive as high efficient adsorbents to remove arsenic [15], nickel [16], and lead [17], for example.

Recent studies have shown that some filtration materials such as sand and burned clay coated with oxides (oxyhydroxides) of iron, aluminum, or manganese act as good and inexpensive sorbents [18–21].

In the present study, the characteristics of two prepared coated adsorbents, namely, manganese oxide-coated sand and manganese oxide-coated crushed brick, have been investigated.

Thermodynamic and kinetic studies of phosphorus ions (PO_4^{3-}) and Pb(II) and Ni(II) ions from aqueous solution adsorption onto these materials were also undertaken. The main objectives of this investigation were to examine quantitatively the effect of contact time, pH, and concentration on the removal of phosphorus ions (PO_4^{3-}) and Pb(II) and Ni(II) ions from aqueous solutions as well as to check in detail the kinetics of the phosphorus ions (PO_4^{3-}) and Pb(II) and Ni(II) ions from aqueous solution and ion-removal process.

2. Materials and methods

2.1 Sample preparation

In our previous works [20, 21], the average diameter for sand and crushed brick grains was 0.6–0.7 and 0.9–1.2 mm, respectively [20, 21], and the specific gravities were 2.50 and 2.39 g/cm^3 for sand and crushed brick, respectively [20, 21].

The manganese oxide-coated adsorbents (MOCS, sand, and MOCB, crushed brick) were prepared by impregnation according to the procedure proposed by Bajpai and Chaudhuri and adopted in our previous research work [20–22].

Before MnO_2 impregnation, an acidic purification procedure (acid wash with 1 M HCl) [20, 21, 23] was made to the adsorbents to remove impurities, which could affect the adsorption results. The reaction of $KMnO_4$ with hot $MnCl_2$ solution (48–50°C) under alkaline conditions (pH 9) over a period of 48 h [20] was the favorable conditions to ensure the application of the MnO_2 coating on the two adsorbent surfaces.

2.2 Chemicals

To prepare aqueous solutions containing phosphates and metal ions at various concentrations, sodium phosphate salt (NaH_2PO_4), lead nitrate salt [$Pb(NO_3)_2$], and nickel chloride salt ($NiCl_2$_$6H_2O$, analytical grade) solutions were used. The initial pH values of the solutions were adjusted by adding either nitric acid or sodium hydroxide solution [20, 21].

All chemicals used for the pre-treatment of the adsorbents, as well as for the adsorption tests, were of analytical grade (HCl, $MnCl_2$, $KMnO_4$, NaOH, HNO_3).

A calibrated pH meter (model pH 540 GLP) equipped with a combined glass electrode (SENTIX 41) [20, 21] was used to ensure the measurements of pH.

2.3 Sorbent characterization

X-ray diffractometer (Siemens, Germany) with Cu Kα radiation (λ = 0.154 nm) was used to determine the mineralogy of the manganese oxide-coating sorbents. The single-point BET (N_2) adsorption procedure was employed to characterize the specific surface area (m^2/g) of each adsorbent before and after coating [20, 21].

The pH of the point of zero charge (pHpzc) was determined by adding 0.1 g of adsorbent to a series of bottles that contained 50 ml of deionizer water. The pH of each solution was adjusted in the range of 1.0–9.0 by the addition of either 0.1 M HNO_3 or 0.1 M NaOH solutions. The bottles were then rotated for 1 h in a shaker and the pH values of the contents measured at the end of the test. The pH values of the suspensions were plotted as a function of the initial pH of the solutions, the resulting curve theoretically crossing the bisector of the axes at the point of zero charge [20, 21]. It is to note that the pHpzc values of 4.5 and 4.3 were obtained for MOCS and MOCB, respectively.

Philips XL 30 scanning electron microscope (SEM) was used to describe the morphology of the adsorbents before and after coating, and elemental spectra were obtained using energy-dispersive X-ray spectroscopy during the SEM observations [20, 21].

2.4 Adsorption experiments

The two prepared materials were first used in batch experiments to check the effect of the initial metal ion concentration on the adsorption kinetics and the influence of the initial pH. Five grams of manganese oxide-coated sorbent was added to 250 ml of each ion solution of known initial concentration [20, 21] and was used for the kinetic studies. The initial pH was adjusted to 5 with dilute HNO_3 or NaOH solution. Prepared solutions were shaken continuously for 4 h at the desired temperature (10, 20, and 40°C). This experiment was released by using a thermostatically controlled shaking water bath. Samples were taken at various time intervals and were immediately vacuum-filtered through a 0.45-μm membrane filter [20, 21].

Atomic absorption spectrophotometry (Hitachi Z-6100) was used to determine the residual ion concentration in each filtrate. Five percent was estimated to be the analytical errors. To ensure the veracity of the experimental results, all experiments were duplicated [20, 21].

To understand the influence of pH on the considered ion adsorption, experiments were performed at various initial pH values within the range 2–7 with the initial Pb(II) ion concentration being maintained at 50 mg/l and from 2 to 11 for Ni(II) and PO_4^{3-} ions. For each test, 1 g of sorbent was added to 25 ml of all considered ion solution, with the suspensions being shaken for 4 h at 20 ± 1°C [20, 21].

2.5 Adsorption isotherms

2.5.1 Isotherm determination

Experiments were conducted at 10°C, 20°C, and 40°C, respectively. At each temperature, 5 g of sorbent were contacted for 4 h with 250 ml of ion solution of different initial concentration [20, 21]. The adsorption equilibrium data were analyzed in terms of the Langmuir and Freundlich isotherm models. The linear forms of the Langmuir and Freundlich isotherms [24] may be expressed, respectively, by the following equations [20, 21]:

$$Ce/qe = 1/q_0b + Ce/q_0 \quad (1)$$

$$\log q_e = \log K_F + \frac{1}{n} \log C_e \quad (2)$$

where the Langmuir isotherm constants are q_0 (mmol/g) and b (g/mmol) and the Freundlich isotherm constants are K_F and n. The measure of the adsorption capacity of the sorbent value is q_0 (maximum amount of ions adsorbed at the temperature under consideration) [20, 21].

2.5.2 Determination of thermodynamic adsorption parameters

The standard Gibbs free energy (ΔG^0), the standard enthalpy (ΔH^0), and the standard entropy (ΔS^0) were determined to explain the effect of temperature on the adsorption parameters. It is known that the adsorption of metal ions is a reversible process corresponding to a heterogeneous equilibrium. The Gibbs free energy (ΔG^0) was determined from the following relationship [25, 26]:

$$\Delta G_0 = RT \ln K_L \quad (3)$$

with R being the gas constant, K_L being equilibrium constant obtained from the Langmuir equation, and T being the absolute temperature (K). The enthalpy change (ΔH^0) and the entropy change (ΔS^0) were evaluated from Van't Hoff's equation:

$$\log K_L = \frac{\Delta S^o}{2.303R} - \frac{\Delta H^o}{2.303RT} \quad (4)$$

The values of ΔH^0 and ΔS^0 were calculated from the slope and intercept of the Van't Hoff plot of log K_L versus 1/T.

The Gibbs free energy

$$\Delta G^0 = \Delta H^0 - T\Delta S^0 \quad (5)$$

indicates the degree of spontaneity of the adsorption process, with a higher negative value reflecting a more energetically favorable adsorption process.

2.5.3 Kinetic parameters of adsorption

In order to analyze the ion adsorption kinetics onto MOCS and MOCB, three kinetic models including the pseudo-first-order equation [27], the pseudo-second-order equation [28], and the intraparticle diffusion model [29] were applied to the experimental data obtained for the time-dependent ion adsorption.

The pseudo-first-order kinetic model is given by the equation:

$$\log(q_e - q_t) = \log q_e - \frac{k_1 t}{2.303} \quad (6)$$

Similarly, the pseudo-second-order kinetic model may be written as.

$$\frac{t}{q_t} = \frac{1}{k_2 q_e^2} + \frac{t}{q_e} \quad (7)$$

while the intraparticle diffusion model may be written as:

$$qt = ktt1/2 + C \quad (8)$$

qe and qt are the amounts of solute adsorbed per unit mass of adsorbent (mmol/g) at equilibrium and at any given time t, respectively; the pseudo-first-order rate constant for the adsorption process (min^{-1}) is k_1; the rate constant for the pseudo-second-order adsorption process [g/(mmol min)] is k_2; the initial adsorption rate for the pseudo-second order adsorption process [mmol/(g min)] is k_2qe_2 = h; the intraparticle diffusion rate constant [mmol/(g min)] is kt; and C is a constant. Linear plots of log(qe − qt) versus t, t/qt versus t, and qt versus t1/2 suggest the applicability of the kinetic models to the system under consideration. The kinetic parameters can be determined from the slopes and intercepts of these plots.

2.6 Determination of the activation energy

The activation energy for all considered ion adsorption was calculated via the Arrhenius Equation [26]:

$$k = k_0 \exp.(-Ea/RT) \tag{9}$$

where k is the rate constant, k_0 [g/(mmol min)] is a temperature-independent factor, Ea (J/mol) is the activation energy of the adsorption process, R is the gas constant [8.314 J/(mol K)], and T is the adsorption temperature (K). The linear form of Eq. (9) is as follows:

$$\ln k = -Ea/RT + \ln k_0 \tag{10}$$

When ln k is plotted versus 1/T, a straight line of slope –Ea/R is obtained. In our case, the rate constant under consideration was k_2, i.e., relating to the pseudo-second-order model.

3. Results and discussion

3.1 Sorbent characterization

3.1.1 SEM micrographs and EDAX spectra

To observe the morphology of the uncoated and the manganese oxide-coated sand (MOCS) and manganese oxide-coated crushed brick (MOCB), SEM micrographs were taken. Obtained results from SEM images of acid-washed uncoated sand (US) and crushed brick (UB) (**Figure 1(a)** and **(c)**) showed that the US surface was characterized by a very ordered silica crystals, and for UB it was principally a regular aluminosilicate. The surfaces of the two virgin materials seem to be uniform and smooth with small cracks and light roughness, but these manganese-oxide-coated surfaces (MOCS **Figure 1(b)**, MOCB **Figure 1(d)**) were covered by newborn manganese oxides that were certainly obtained during the coating process. **Figure 1(b)** and **(d)** also showed manganese oxides formed in clusters, apparently on occupied surfaces. The amount of manganese on the surface of the MOCS and MOCB was determined by acid digestion analysis. Results obtained for the Mn deposits were approximately 1.5 mg Mn/g for sand and 2 mg Mn/g for crushed brick. It is to note also that the quantity of manganese deposit obtained in this work for the two sorbents was found to be higher than that generally mentioned in the literature, which is about 0.003–0.5 mg Mn/g of sand [28, 30]. This reflects the effectiveness of the coating process used in this study.

The X-ray diffraction (XRD) patterns of the two coated sorbents (data not shown) revealed that the manganese oxides were amorphous, since no specific diffraction ray indicative of any specific crystalline phase was detected.

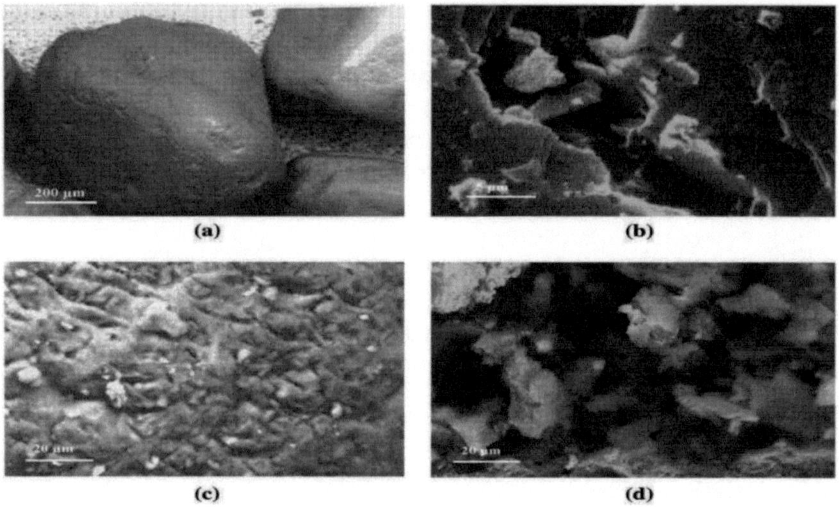

Figure 1.
SEM micrographs of samples: (a) US, (b) MOCS, (c) uncoated crushed brick, and (d) MOCB.

Figure 2(a) of the EDAX spectra of MOCS shows that Mn, O, and Si are the main constituents. These had been expected to be the principal elements of MOCS. In fact, EDAX the important peak of Si occurring in EDAX spectrum was apparently related to the too thin coating, or manganese oxides did not cover the full surface of the MOCS, allowing the X-ray to reach the sand support. From the EDAX spectrum of MOCB illustrated in **Figure 2(b)**, it was shown that Mn, O, Si, Al, Ca, and K are the dominant constituents. The presence of the Mn peak indicates the effectiveness of the adopted coating process.

3.1.2 Specific surface area

It is to note that specific surface areas of the two sorbents increased after coating. The obtained values of surface area were 1.36 and 1.86 m^2/g, for uncoated sand and uncoated crushed brick, respectively, after coating with manganese oxide the surface area of sorbents increased to 3.81 and 4.64 m^2/g, respectively. We can conclude that the addition of the manganese oxides contributes to the increase in both inner and surface porosities.

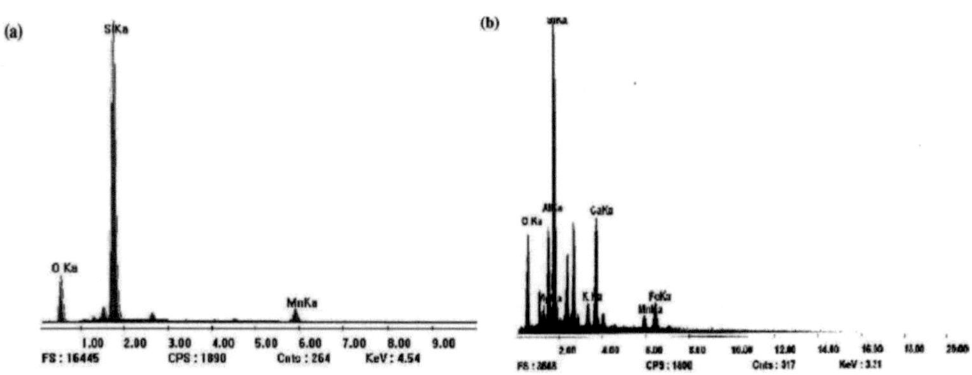

Figure 2.
EDAX spectrum of (a) MOCS and (b) MOCB.

3.2 Batch adsorption experiments

3.2.1 Kinetic study

To study the effect of contact time on the sorption of all different ions, a different initial concentration was used: 10 mg/l and 50 mg/l for PO_4^{3-} and for Pb(II) and Ni(II), respectively, and a fixed pH solution of 5.0. The data showed that the sorption on MOCB and MOCS was very fast at the initial stages of the contact period, and thereafter it becomes slower near the equilibrium. The difference between the surface areas of each adsorbent can explain the differences in their sorption capacities. The sorption of all elements on the two sorbents was very fast too in the first few minutes and sharply reached a 80% removal after only 10–15 min. When the sorption process approached completion, the sorption slowed down. In this work, subsequent experiments were carried out at a contact time of 2 h for all sorbents to ensure that the equilibrium time was practically attained (**Figure 3**).

3.2.2 Effect of initial pH

Adsorption process is strongly related to pH and to the charge on both the adsorbate and the adsorbent. The surface charge on a manganese oxide surface varies with the solution pH due to the exchange of H+ ions. The surface groups on manganese oxide are amphoteric and can act as either an acid or a base. Consequently, the oxide surface can undergo protonation and deprotonation in response to changes in the solution pH [20].

The optimal pH was obtained at around pH 4. It is to note that the removal decreases continuously for pH values ranging between around 4 and 10 according to other works dealing with sorption of phosphate ions on hematite and Al_2O_3 [31], ion-exchange fiber [32], alunite [33], and bauxite [34]. The decrease in the phosphate ion uptake, occurring beyond pH 5, could be probably attributed in one hand to a competition between phosphate ions and hydroxyl ions for the sorption on the surface Lewis acid sites of the sorbent [21] and in another hand by considering a zero point of charge of the sorbent. In fact, above the zero point of charge, the positive charge density on the surface of the sorbents increases which disfavors the sorption of phosphate ions. The sorption of phosphate onto hydroxylated mineral surface can be described by a ligand exchange mechanism [35, 36], which causes an increase in pH due to the hydroxyl ions released from the oxidic sorbent. Concerning nickel sorption is negligible at the low pH values probably due to the competition effects between H_3O^+ ion and the considered species while increases progressively from pH 4. A maximum is reached at around pH 7–8; then, above pH 8 the amount of adsorbed nickel decreases as the pH increases. According to the simple species, diagrams, which were constructed for Ni(II), up to pH 8, nickel is present in the

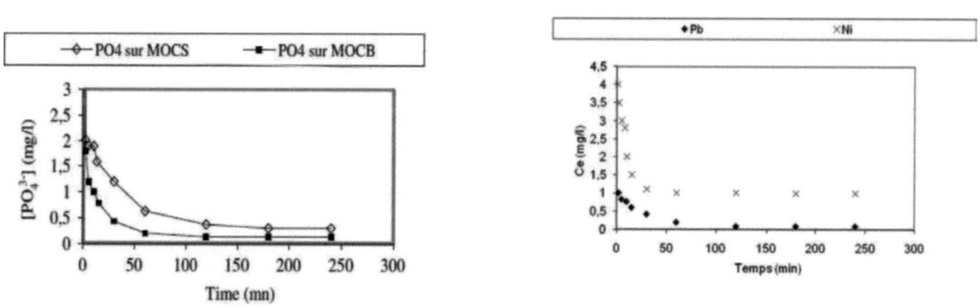

Figure 3.
Effect of contact time on all considered ions removal at pH 5 onto (a) phosphorus ions and (b) lead and nickel ions.

solution mainly in the form of Ni^{2+} ions. Neutral $Ni(OH)_2$ particles start to precipitate at pH 8 and become predominant at pH 11 [37].

The adsorption of Pb(II) ions onto both adsorbents was markedly dependent on the pH value. When the initial solution pH increased from 2 to 7, the removal of Pb (II) ion was possibly inhibited following the competition between metal ions and H+ for the available adsorption locations, while the uptake of H+ ions was more preponderant. However, the adsorption of Pb (II) ions increased with the deprotonation of the binding sites caused by the negative charge density of each adsorbent and this with the increase of the pH [20].

From our previous work [20], we have attributed this increase in adsorption with decreasing H+ ion concentration (relatively high pH values), which indicates that ion exchange is one of the major adsorption processes. Due to the equal of positive and negative groups, the total surface charge is zero, which can explain the effect of pH in terms of pHpzc value of the adsorbent. The pHpzc of MOCS and MOCB was investigated and determined to be 4.5 and 4.3, respectively [20]. If the pH was below the pHpzc, the surface charge on the adsorbent was positive; however when it is above the pHpzc value, the surface charge was negative, so the two considered adsorbents (MOCS and MOCB) have positive surface charge, and this is below the respective pH values of 4.3 and 4.5; therefore, the absorption of Pb (II) ions was low. However, the surface charges of the two adsorbents MOCS and MOCB were negative when the pH was increased above 4.3 and 4.5, respectively. The uptake is going to increase if the Pb (II) species count were either neutral or positively charged. Also, at higher pH values than pHpzc, the cation removal would be favored, and for anion, the adsorption was favored at pH values lower than pHpzc.

3.3 Sorption isotherm

The sorption of all considered ions increases as its initial concentration in the solution increases, until a maximum value (saturation state) is reached.

The maximum sorption capacity, Q_0, calculated from the Langmuir equation at 20°C, is indicated in **Table 1**.

As seen, sorption on the two coated sorbents is greater than that on virgin sand. The coatings significantly increase adsorption capacity, resulting in higher interactions between sorbents and sorbate. The values of sorption constants, derived from the Freundlich model (**Table 2**), show that the KF constant—which is a measure of sorption capacity—remains higher for MOCB than for MOCS. Values obtained of $1 < n < 10$ imply favorable sorption of all ions on the two sorbents [20, 21].

3.4 Thermodynamic adsorption parameters

Thermodynamic parameters were evaluated using the data obtained at the temperatures of 10, 20, and 40 °C. The values of ΔG0 were calculated using the

Element	SCM			BCM		
	Q_0 (mg/g)	b (l/mg)	R^2	Q_0 (mg/g)	b (l/mg)	R^2
Lead	6	2.56	0.98	6.25	3.36	0.97
Phosphate ions	1.96	0.41	0.97	2.08	1.38	0.98
Nickel	3.33	0.34	0.99	3.7	0.62	0.99

Table 1.
Langmuir parameters.

Langmuir isotherm constant, b. The values of ΔH^0 and ΔS^0 were obtained from the slope and intercept of the plot of ln b versus 1/T. **Table 3** illustrates the calculated parameters for the two adsorbents. The spontaneous nature of all ions adsorption by the two adsorbents was confirmed by the negative values of ΔG^0. On the contrary, positive values of ΔH^0 show that the adsorption process was endothermic in nature, while the positive values of ΔS^0 show the increasing randomness at solid/liquid interface during the adsorption process.

3.5 Determination of kinetic parameters

The pseudo-first-order and pseudo-second-order kinetic equations as well as the intraparticle diffusion model were applied to predict the kinetics of the adsorption of all ions onto the two adsorbents. The values, which are founded for the kinetic model, were excessively high (> 0.998); this result decreases for the intraparticle

Element	SCM			BCM		
	K_f	1/n	R^2	K_f	1/n	R^2
Lead	3.53	0.26	0.997	2.97	0.33	0.97
Phosphate ions	0.58	0.39	0.98	0.78	0.36	0.98
Nickel	0.32	0.22	0.98	0.61	0.26	0,91

Table 2.
Freundlich parameters.

Temperature (°C)			10	20	40
MOCS	Lead	ΔG° (kJ/mol)	−30.948	−32.042	−34.229
		ΔH° (kJ/mol)	42.776	42.776	42.776
		ΔS° (kJ/(kmol))	0.252	0.252	0.252
	Nickel	ΔG° (kJ/mol)	−23.35	−24.17	−25.82
		ΔH° (kJ/mol)	17.63	17.63	17.63
		ΔS° (kJ/(kmol))	0.14	0.14	0.14
	Phosphate ions	ΔG° (kJ/mol)	−24.827	−25.704	−27.459
		ΔH° (kJ/mol)	12.342	12.342	12.342
		ΔS° (kJ/(kmol))	0.129	0.129	0.129
MOCB	Lead	ΔG° (kJ/mol)	−28.432	−29.437	−31.446
		ΔH° (kJ/mol)	32.753	32.753	32.753
		ΔS° (kJ/(kmol))	0.211	0.211	0.211
	Nickel	ΔG° (kJ/mol)	−24.78	−25.68	−27.44
		ΔH° (kJ/mol)	22.78	22.78	22.78
		ΔS° (kJ/(kmol))	0.16	0.16	0.16
	Phosphate ions	ΔG° (kJ/mol)	−27.703	−28.862	−30.640
		ΔH° (kJ/mol)	24.693	24.693	24.693
		ΔS° (kJ/(kmol))	0.182	0.182	0.182

Table 3.
Thermodynamic parameters.

diffusion equation and also for the pseudo-first-order equation. Furthermore, the quantity of all considered elements adsorption at equilibrium (qe) compared to the experimental data concluded the pseudo-second-order link was more reasonable than that of the pseudo-first order model. This proposed that the removal operation move forward via a pseudo-second-order rather than a pseudo-first-order kinetic model. For this model, the initial adsorption rate, h, and the rate constant K2 diminished with the increase of the initial concentration of all considered ions; then, a limiting step may involve chemisorption [20].

4. Conclusions

Results obtained from this work showed that the deposited oxides were essentially amorphous and corresponded to 1.5 mg Mn(II)/g sand and 2 mg Mn(II)/g crushed brick.

The optimal pH adsorption for all considered ions was 5, and adsorption capacities were higher onto MOCB than MOCS.

The activation energy values for the two adsorbents found from Arrhenius plots and the kinetics which found pseudo-second order suggested that the limiting step of adsorption of all ions could be chemisorption. The results obtained in the present study suggest that manganese oxide-coated adsorbents are potentially suitable for removing of cations and anions from aqueous solution.

Author details

Nesrine Boujelben
Water Energy and Environment Laboratory, Geology Department, National Engineering School of Sfax, Sfax, Tunisia

*Address all correspondence to: nesrine.boujelben@tunet.tn

IntechOpen

© 2020 The Author(s). Licensee IntechOpen. This chapter is distributed under the terms of the Creative Commons Attribution License (http://creativecommons.org/licenses/by/3.0), which permits unrestricted use, distribution, and reproduction in any medium, provided the original work is properly cited. CC BY

References

[1] Rao MM, Rao GPC, Seshaiah K, Choudary NV, Wang MC. Activated carbon from Ceiba pentandra hulls, an agricultural waste, as an adsorbent in the removal of lead and zinc from aqueous solutions. Waste Management (Oxford). 2008;**28**(5):849-858

[2] Liu Z, Zhong X, Wang Y, Ding Z, Wang C, Wang G, et al. An efficient adsorption of manganese oxides/activated carbon composite for lead(II) ions from aqueous solution. Arabian Journal for Science and Engineering. 2018;**43**:2155-2165

[3] Sreejalekshmi KG, Krishnan KA, Anirudhan TS. Adsorption of Pb(II) and Pb(II)-citric acid on sawdust activated carbon: Kinetic and equilibrium isotherm studies. Journal of Hazardous Materials. 2009;**161**(2-3):1506-1513

[4] Aziz HA, Adlan MN, Ariffin KS. Heavy metals (Cd, Pb, Zn, Ni, Cu and Cr(III)) removal from water in Malaysia: Post treatment by high quality limestone. Bioresource Technology. 2008;**99**(6):1578-1583

[5] Liu YX, Yan JM, Yuan DX, Li QL, Wu XY. The study of lead removal from aqueous solution using an electrochemical method with a stainless steel net electrode coated with single wall carbon nanotubes. Chemical Engineering Journal. 2013;**218**:81-88

[6] Al-Othman ZA, Naushad Inamuddin M. Organic–inorganic type composite cation exchanger poly-o-toluidine Zr(IV) tungstate: Preparation, physicochemical characterization and its analytical application in separation of heavy metals. Chemical Engineering Journal. 2011;**172**(1):369-375

[7] O'Connell DW, Birkinshaw C, O'Dwyer TF. Heavy metal adsorbents prepared from the modification of cellulose: A review. Bioresource Technology. 2008;**99**:6709-6724

[8] Mohan D, Singh KP. Single- and multi-component adsorption of cadmium and zinc using activated carbon derived from bagasse—An agricultural waste. Water Research. 2002;**36**(9):2304-2318

[9] Han RP, Zhu L, Zou WH, Wang DT, Shi J, Yang JJ. Removal of copper(II) and lead(II) from aqueous solution by manganese oxide coated sand—II. Equilibrium study and competitive adsorption. Journal of Hazardous Materials. 2006;**137**(1):480-488

[10] Ghaedi M, Biyareh MN, Kokhdan SN, Shamsaldini S, Sahraei R, Daneshfar A, et al. Comparison of the efficiency of palladium and silver nanoparticles loaded on activated carbon and zinc oxide nanorods loaded on activated carbon as new adsorbents for removal of Congo red from aqueous solution: Kinetic and isotherm study. Materials Science and Engineering: C. 2012;**32**(4):725-734

[11] Sun YB, Yang SB, Chen Y, Ding CC, Cheng WC, Wang XK. Adsorption and desorption of U(VI) on functionalized graphene oxides: A combined experimental and theoretical study. Environmental Science & Technology. 2015;**49**:4255-4262

[12] Ma MH, Gao HY, Sun YB, Huang MS. The adsorption and desorption of Ni(II) on Al substituted goethite. Journal of Molecular Liquids. 2015;**201**:30-35. International Journal of Environmental Research Public Health. 2017, 14, 1145 10 of 11

[13] Sounthararajah DP, Loganathan P, Kandasamy J, Vigneswaran S. Effects of humic acid and suspended solids on the removal of heavy metals from water by adsorption onto granular activated carbon. International Journal of Environmental Research and Public Health. 2015;**12**:10475-10489

[14] Lee SM, Laldawngliana C, Tiwari D. Iron oxide nano-particles-immobilized-sand material in the treatment of Cu(II), Cd(II) and Pb(II) contaminated waste waters. Chemical Engineering Journal. 2012;**195**:103-111

[15] Tani Y, Miyata N, Ohashi M, Ohnuki T, Seyama H, Iwahori K, et al. Interaction of inorganic arsenic with biogenic manganese oxide produced by a Mn-oxidizing fungus, strain KR21-2. Environmental Science & Technology. 2004;**38**:6618-6624

[16] Kennedy C, Smith DS, Warren LA. Surface chemistry and relative Ni sorptive capacities of synthetic hydrous Mn oxyhydroxides under variable wetting and drying regimes. Geochimica et Cosmochimica Acta. 2004;**68**:443-454

[17] Villalobos M, Bargar J, Sposito G. Mechanisms of Pb(II) sorption on a biogenic manganese oxide. Environmental Science & Technology. 2005;**39**:569-576

[18] Benjamin MM, Slatten RS, Bailey RP, Bennett T. Sorption and filtration of metals using iron oxide coated sand. Water Research. 1996;**30**:2609-2620

[19] Sharma SK, Petrusevski B, Schippers JC. Characterisation of coated sand from iron removal plants. Journal of Water Supply: Research and Technology. 2002;**2**:247-257

[20] Boujeben N, Bouzid J, Elouear Z. Removal of Lead(II) ions from aqueous solutions using manganese oxide-coated adsorbents: Characterization and kinetic study. Adsorption Science & Technology. 2009;**27**:2

[21] Boujelben N, Bouhamed F, Elouear Z, Bouzid J, Feki M. Removal of phosphorus ions from aqueous solutions using manganese-oxide-coated sand and brick. Desalination and Water Treatment. 2014;**52**:2282-2292

[22] Bajpai S, Chaudhuri M. Removal of arsenic from ground water by manganese dioxide–coated sand. Journal of Environmental Engineering. 1999;**125**(8):782-784

[23] Lo SL, Jengh T, Lai CH. Characteristics and adsorption properties of an ironcoated sand. Water Science and Technology. 1997;**35**:63-70

[24] Seader JD, Herley EJ. Separation Process Principles. New York: Wiley; 1998

[25] Aksu Z. Determination of the equilibrium, kinetic and thermodynamic parameters of the batch biosorption of nickel (II) ions onto chlorella vulgaris. Process Biochemistry. 2002;**38**(1):89-99

[26] Namasivayam C, Ranganathan K. Waste Fe(III)/Cr(III) hydroxide as adsorbent for the removal of Cr(VI) from aqueous solution and chromium plating industry waste water. Environmental Pollution. 1993;**82**:255-261

[27] Panday KK, Prasad G, Singh VN. Copper(II) removal from aqueous solutions by fly ash. Water Research. 1985;**19**:869-873

[28] Selvaraj R, Younghun K, Cheol KJ. Removal of copper from aqueous solution by aminated and protonated mesoporous aluminas: Kinetics and equilibrium. Journal of Colloid and Interface Science. 2004;**273**:14-21

[29] Chiron N, Guilet R, Deydier E. Adsorption of Cu(II) and Pb(II) onto a grafted silica: Isotherms and kinetic models. Water Research. 2003;**37**(13):3079-3086

[30] Chang YY, Kim KS, Jung JH, Yang JK, Lee SM. Application of iron-coated sand and manganese-coated sand on the treatment of both As(III) and

As(V). Water Science and Technology. 2007;**55**:69-75

[31] Hu P-Y, Hsieh Y-H, Chen J-C, Chang C-Y. Characteristics of manganese-coated sand using SEM and EDAX analysis. Journal of Colloid and Interface Science. 2004;**274**:308-312

[32] Horanyi G, Joo P. Some peculiarities in the specific adsorption of phosphate ions on hematite c-Al_2O_3 as reflected by radiotracer studies. Journal of Colloid and Interface Science. 2002;**247**:12-17

[33] Xia LR, Jinlong G, Hongxiao T. Adsorption of fluoride, phosphate, and arsenate ions on a new type of ion exchange fiber. Journal of Colloid and Interface Science. 2002;**248**:268-274

[34] Ozacar M. Phosphate adsorption characteristics of alunite to be used as a cement additive. Cement and Concrete Research. 2003;**2372**:1-5

[35] Altundogan HS, Tumen F. Removal of phosphates from aqueous solutions by using bauxite. I: Effect of pH on the adsorption of various phosphates. Journal of Chemical Technology & Biotechnology. 2001;**77**:77-85

[36] Goldberg S, Sposito G. On the mechanism of specific phosphate adsorption by hydroxylated mineral surfaces: A review. Communications in Soil Science and Plant Analysis. 1985;**16**:801-821

[37] Mavros P, Zouboulis AI, Lazaridis NK. Removal of metal ions from wastewaters the case of nickel. Journal of Environmental Technology. 1993;**14**:83-91

Chapter 3

A Role for Heavy Metal Toxicity and Air Pollution in Respiratory Tract Cancers

Chanda Siddoo-Atwal

Abstract

Cigarette smoke and air pollution have been associated with lung cancer and naso pharyngeal and laryngeal cancer, respectively. Significant concentrations of select heavy metals including lead and cadmium have been isolated in popular cigarette brands, and these heavy metals can be inhaled via smoking. Lead is able to mimic the activity of calcium in the human body, thereby leading to toxic effects in a variety of target organs. Lead perturbs and alters the release of intracellular calcium stores from organelles like the endoplasmic reticulum (ER) and mitochondria. A rise in mitochondrial calcium stimulates the generation of reactive oxygen species (ROS) and free fatty acids which can further promote calcium release and, ultimately, result in cell death. In the case of cadmium, the renal proximal tubule of the kidney accumulates freely filtered and metallothionein-bound metal, which is degraded in endosomes and lysosomes. This results in the release of free cadmium into the cytosol where it can generate reactive oxygen species and activate cell death pathways. In developing countries, indoor air pollution due to the domestic use of unprocessed biomass fuels such as wood, dung, and coal is another cause of respiratory tract cancers in humans. In some developed countries such as Australia and Canada, the alarming increase in forest fire frequency due to climate change and the associated smoke released into the environment is also likely to pose a future human health risk. Polycyclic organic particles in biomass and forest fire smoke can include carcinogens such as benzo[a]pyrene, which is also found in cigarette smoke. Benzo[a]pyrene can induce apoptosis in mammalian cells by initiating mitochondrial dysfunction, activating the intrinsic caspase pathway (caspase-3 and caspase-9), and via p53 activation. The constitutive activation of apoptotic pathways has been linked to carcinogenesis in a number of cancer models.

Keywords: cigarette smoke, indoor and outdoor air pollution, lead, cadmium, benzo[a]pyrene, respiratory tract cancers

1. Introduction

"Smoking is hazardous to the health" is a phrase that is commonly used and understood in many parts of the world. In actuality, "smoke" is the hazard. The inhalation of smoke from cigarettes, indoor air pollution, and forest fires currently constitutes a serious public health issue of increasing importance as environmental conditions rapidly change on the planet.

The presence of heavy metals and other toxic and trace elements in tobacco smoke is a major concern. Notably, lead (Pb), arsenic (As), chromium (Cr), nickel (Ni), and cadmium (Cd) are usually associated with its adverse health effects. Heavy metals can pass from tobacco to the smoke and smoke condensate [1]. Although cigarette filters remove a portion of these elements, environmental smoke pollution occurs via the smoke exhaled by the smoker and the sidestream smoke emitted by the burning cigarette. The sidestream smoke inhaled by non-smokers can contain a relatively high concentration of heavy metals. This process of passive smoking can result in the deposition of heavy metals deep in the lung tissue [2].

Lead and cadmium, particularly, both of which have long half-lives (10–12 years), accumulate in tissues and fluids following smoke exposure. Biomonitoring studies reveal that smokers have substantially higher lead and cadmium levels than nonsmokers. Bioaccumulation of metals has also been demonstrated in nonsmokers, who are chronically exposed to secondhand smoke [3]. Smoking-related diseases can be attributed to the inhalation of many different toxins including heavy metals. Heavy metals like lead have been shown to affect various biochemical processes in the human body including calcium metabolism and the activation of cell death pathways which are involved in carcinogenesis [4].

A significant percentage of people in developing countries utilize coal and biomass fuels like wood and dung for domestic energy. These materials are often burnt in simple stoves resulting in incomplete combustion. Consequently, women and young children are exposed to high levels of indoor air pollution daily. Many substances in biomass smoke are hazardous to the health including carbon monoxide, nitrous oxides, sulfur oxides (principally from coal), formaldehyde, and polycyclic organic matter (notably carcinogens such as benzo[a]pyrene [BaP]). Particles, particularly with diameters below 10 microns (PM10), especially those less than 2.5 microns in diameter (PM2.5), can penetrate deeply into the lungs to cause damage to these delicate organs. Epidemiological evidence suggests that indoor air pollution increases the risk of chronic obstructive pulmonary disease and of acute respiratory infections in childhood, which are the most important cause of death among preschool children in developing nations. Biomass smoke is also associated with low birth weight, increased infant and perinatal mortality, pulmonary tuberculosis, nasopharyngeal and laryngeal cancer, cataracts, and lung cancer (specifically, in the case of coal) [5].

The incidence of forest fires is strongly linked to climatic conditions. In fact, climate change is predicted to affect forests in the following ways: increased growth rates, tree-line movements, changes to forest species assemblages, increased fire incidence, more severe droughts in some areas, increased storm damage, and increased insect and pathogen damage [6]. Specifically, predicted impacts of climate change in Australia include increased fuel loadings, drier fuels, and increased dangerous fire weather [7, 8]. Model predictions for Canada have found expectations of decreased fire frequency in parts of the eastern boreal forest, while dramatic increases are expected elsewhere in the country [9]. In fact, over recent decades, the area burned by wildland fires in Canada has steadily increased and is predicted to double by the end of the century accompanied by an increase in length of the fire season [10]. At the same time, it is important to note that several climatic and non-climatic factors besides increased temperatures determine forest fire frequency including ignition sources, fuel loads, vegetation characteristics, rainfall, humidity, wind, topography, landscape fragmentation, and management policies [11]. Currently, research on the health effects of forest and wild fire smoke

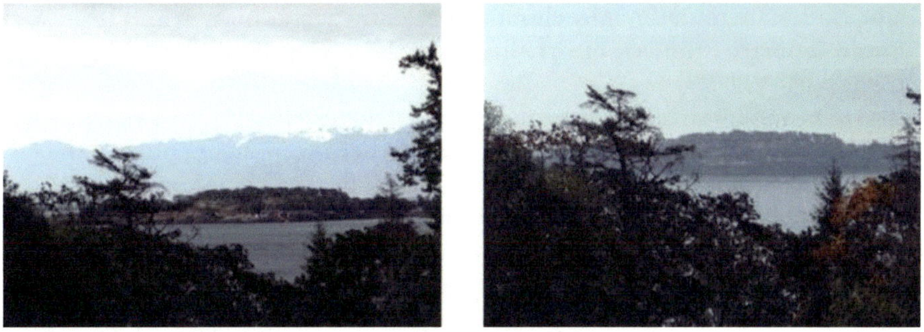

Figure 1.
The same view of the Olympic Mountains in Washington State, USA, before (left) and during (right) forest fire season (2018) in British Columbia, Canada.

is limited [12]. However, smoke from these conflagrations contains the same kind of particles as indoor combustion from wood smoke. Similar to the situation of indoor air pollution from biomass smoke, forest fires generate polycyclic aromatic hydrocarbons (PAHs), which can include carcinogens such as benzo(a)pyrene [BaP] [13]. Polycyclic aromatic hydrocarbons (PAH) like BaP can stimulate various biochemical processes in the body including the continuous activation of apoptotic (cell death) pathways that have been linked to the initiation of carcinogenesis [14]. It is of interest that this chemical compound (BaP) is also found in cigarette smoke (**Figure 1**).

2. Lead [Pb]

Generally, elemental lead use and exposure have decreased significantly since the 1970s due to the innovation of unleaded gasoline and lead-free plumbing and paints. However, lead poisoning is still a serious problem. Lead is very toxic and specifically targets the kidneys, liver, central nervous system, hematopoietic system, and endocrine and reproductive systems. It can be absorbed by women during pregnancy and transferred to the developing fetus. Prenatal lead exposure has been linked to reduced birth weight, preterm delivery, and neurodevelopmental abnormalities in offspring. Exposure occurs mostly as a result of deteriorating house paints, contact at the workplace, hobbies, leaching from lead-containing vessels into food and water, cigarette smoke, and the use of lead in certain traditional medicines and cosmetics. Routes of exposure mainly include inhalation of lead-containing dust particles and ingestion of lead-contaminated food and water [15]. Lead has been classed as a probable carcinogen by the Environmental Protection Agency (EPA) and other regulatory agencies [16, 17].

Lead is able to mimic the activity of calcium in the human body, thereby leading to toxic effects in a variety of target organs [15]. These biochemical effects include the calcium-dependent inhibition of release of several neurotransmitters [18] and augmentation of calcium-dependent events involving protein kinase C and calmodulin [19, 20]. Lead can also be incorporated into the human skeleton instead of calcium.

Moreover, lead perturbs and alters the release of intracellular calcium stores from organelles like the endoplasmic reticulum (ER) and mitochondria [19, 21]. Mitochondria can accumulate large amounts of calcium, for example, in the presence of inorganic phosphate. The rise in calcium results in an upregulation of energy metabolism and an increase in mitochondrial membrane potential. Then, the release of this accumulated calcium through a special channel, permeability transition pore (PTP), can cause mitochondrial depolarization. According to the model of glutamate toxicity, mitochondrial calcium accumulation and resultant membrane depolarization are clearly linked to the initiation of a cell death pathway in mitochondria [22, 23].

A rise in mitochondrial calcium also stimulates the generation of reactive oxygen species (ROS) and free fatty acids which can further promote opening of the PTP, resulting in calcium release and, ultimately, in cell death [23]. Many genes and proteins that respond to conditions of oxidative stress stimulated by ROS release within the cell subsequently trigger apoptosis. Because mitochondria are important regulators of cellular redox status, the induction of oxidative stress exhibits its effects upon these organelles by triggering the intrinsic apoptotic pathway via cytochrome c release and caspase cascade activation [24, 25].

In this regard, it has been reported in various experiments that lead poisoning results in cellular damage mediated by the formation of reactive oxygen species (ROS) [26]. An elevation in the relative activities of certain antioxidant enzymes such as glutathione peroxidase has also been reported in the erythrocytes of lead-exposed workers [27].

In one large epidemiological study in Eastern Europe spanning several years, an elevated risk of renal cell carcinoma was observed in the category of highest cumulative occupational lead exposure [28]. Lead has been found to induce renal tumors in rats and mice [29, 30]. Lead causes DNA strand breakage and 8-hydroxy-deoxyguanosine adduct formation in calf thymus DNA [31]. It induces sister chromatid exchanges in Chinese hamster ovary cells [32]. Lead-induced cytotoxicity and apoptosis have been demonstrated in human cancer cells via various cellular and molecular processes including oxidative stress induction and caspase-3 activation [15]. Finally, mitochondrial alterations appear to play a central role in lead-induced rod photoreceptor cell apoptosis [33].

Taken together, the above data point to the activation of apoptotic pathways as a possible mechanism of lead carcinogenesis. It clearly has the potential to initiate cancer as described in a new approach to cancer risk assessment based on an apoptotic model of tumor formation. In this two-stage model of tumor formation, Step I exposure to a carcinogen (Pb in this case), possibly facilitated by a genetic predisposition, results in an epigenetic or genetic event causing continuous apoptotic activation of cells in the target tissue. In Step II, when the carcinogen may or may not be present, resistance to apoptosis and continuous cell proliferation result due to another genetic or epigenetic event [4, 14].

3. Cadmium [Cd]

Cadmium is a heavy metal that is widely distributed in the earth's crust, while the highest level of cadmium compounds is found in sedimentary rocks and marine phosphates. Human exposure to this element can occur through employment in primary metal industries, eating contaminated food, smoking cigarettes (a major contributor), and working in cadmium-contaminated places. Other sources of cadmium include emissions from mining, smelting, manufacturing batteries, pigments, stabilizers, and alloys. The main routes of cadmium exposure are via inhalation or cigarette smoke and ingestion of food. It is a severe pulmonary and gastrointestinal irritant, which can prove fatal when inhaled or ingested in extreme cases [15].

Cadmium levels in the body can be measured in the blood or urine. Typically, blood and urine cadmium levels are higher in cigarette smokers, intermediate in former smokers, and lower in nonsmokers. The circulatory system is an important distribution route of cadmium toxicity, and blood vessels are considered to be the primary target. Chronic cadmium inhalation exposure is associated with changes in pulmonary function and chest radiographs consistent with emphysema. Chronic low-level cadmium exposure can also cause decreases in olfactory function and bone mineral density and osteoporosis.

Cadmium compounds have been classified as human carcinogens by certain regulatory agencies including the International Agency for Research on Cancer and the US National Toxicology Program based on repeated findings of a correlation between occupational cadmium exposure and lung cancer in humans. In addition, there is strong experimental evidence that the pulmonary system is the main target site for carcinogenesis in rodents [17]. Such rodent studies reveal that chronic cadmium inhalation results in pulmonary adenocarcinomas. Oral cadmium exposure in rats is also associated with tumors of the prostate, testes, and hematopoietic system [34–36].

Cadmium is a weak mutagen and the mechanisms of its toxicity are poorly understood. It has been reported to affect signal transduction pathways, induce inositol phosphate formation, increase cytosolic free calcium levels in a variety of cell types, and block calcium channels. At lower micromolar concentrations, cadmium can induce the expression of antioxidant enzymes such as glutathione transferases and metallothioneins suggesting that it causes cellular damage via the generation of ROS, which can initiate DNA damage and activate apoptotic pathways.

Specifically, receptor-mediated endocytosis of freely filtered and metallothionein-bound cadmium causes it to accumulate in the renal proximal tubule of the kidney. Following internalization and degradation of metallothionein-cadmium complexes in endosomes and lysosomes in this kidney model, free cadmium is released into the cytosol, where it can generate ROS and activate cell death pathways [37] implicated in cancer.

4. Polycyclic aromatic hydrocarbons [PAHs] and benzo(a)pyrene [BaP]

Polycyclic aromatic hydrocarbons and their derivatives are a major class of organic compounds that are produced as a result of incomplete combustion of fossil fuels and other organic matter. Consequently, they are prevalent in the human environment and include a number of potent carcinogens. Some of the major sources of these emissions are wood and coal burning, automobiles and other fossil-fuel propelled modes of transportation, heat and power plants, and refuse burning. PAHs are not only present in the air, but are found in many common foods and drinking water and form a significant component of tobacco smoke [38].

Levels of PAHs are routinely measured in the atmosphere for air quality assessment, in sediments and mollusks for environmental monitoring, in biological tissues for monitoring of health effects, and in foodstuffs for safety reasons. Gas chromatography is often chosen for analyzing (separating, identifying, and quantifying) PAHs due to the high degree of selectivity and resolution this method provides [39].

PAH-DNA adducts have been compared in the peripheral leukocytes of non-small cell lung cancer patients and in controls. Adduct formation has been found to be significantly higher in lung cancer cases than in controls. Further, in the cancer patients, adducts were more strongly correlated with lung tumor tissue than with non-tumor lung tissue consistent with a genetic susceptibility to lung cancer as a result of adduct-induced DNA damage [40]. More specifically, BPDE-DNA adducts have been observed in the white blood cells of occupationally exposed workers and cigarette smokers. BaP is metabolically activated to its carcinogenic form benzo(*a*) pyrene diol epoxide (BPDE), and this is an important step in BaP carcinogenicity in experimental animal studies [41]. Moreover, using a specially developed assay on peripheral blood lymphocytes, it has been determined that there is a significant association between the level of in vitro BPDE-induced DNA adducts and risk for lung cancer in humans [42]. In another molecular epidemiologic hospital-based study, DNA repair capacity was measured in cultured lymphocytes from lung cancer patients and controls. It cleverly utilized the host-cell reactivation assay with a reporter gene damaged by the known activated tobacco carcinogen, benzo[*a*] pyrene diol epoxide. It was observed that reduced DNA repair capacity was associated with increased risk of lung cancer in a dose-dependent fashion [43]. In addition, the frequency of BPDE-induced chromosomal aberrations is significantly higher in lymphocyte cultures from lung cancer patients than in controls. These chromosomal aberrations tend to be predominantly single chromatid breaks with few exchanges or isochromatid breaks [44].

There is overwhelming evidence in the scientific literature for BaP-induced lung and respiratory tract carcinogenesis in experimental animals. Highly sensitive immunoassays using antiserum specific for benzo(a)pyrene have revealed a dose-related increase in levels of BaP-DNA adducts in the lung tissue of mice and rabbits following intraperitoneal injection with this chemical carcinogen [45]. In the past, respiratory tract tumors have been induced in Syrian golden hamsters following intratracheal injections of benzo(a)pyrene and benzo(a)pyrene-ferric oxide [46, 47]. In fact, BaP-induced lung cancer in mice is so reproducible that it has become a popular model for studying the potential role of natural products in ameliorating the effects of BaP [48]. It is known that lung carcinogenesis can be induced in Swiss albino mice following biweekly treatment with BaP (50 mg/kg b. wt.) over a period of 16 weeks [49]. Supplementation with hesperidin, a naturally occurring flavonoid in citrus fruits, has been reported to have a chemopreventive activity during BaP-induced lung cancer in Swiss albino mice. It appears to attenuate the accompanying loss in tissue antioxidant function and to have an antiproliferative effect as revealed by histopathological analysis involving proliferating cell nuclear antigen (PCNA) immunostaining [50]. In another interesting chemopreventive study, BaP-induced neoplasia of mouse forestomach was inhibited by a principal component of Japanese soy sauce, 4-hydroxy-2(or 5)-ethyl-5(or 2)-methyl-3(2H)-furanone, suggesting that this *Saccharomyces cerevisiae* metabolite is a potent anticarcinogen [51].

In mouse hepatoma cells, treatment with micromolar concentrations of BaP results in caspase-3 activation, followed by apoptosis. However, caspase-3 activity is blocked and BaP-induced apoptosis attenuated by pretreatment of the cells with a specific inhibitor of caspase-3-like proteases, acetyl-Asp-Glu-Val-Asp-aldehyde [52]. It has also been demonstrated that BaP treatment of mouse hepatoma cells causes apoptosis via the catalytic activation of caspase-9, mitochondrial dysfunction including a loss in membrane potential and cytosolic release of cytochrome c, and phosphorylation of p53 (Ser15) [53]. In BaP-treated human Hep3B (p53-null) cells, necrosis is induced at 12 hours and apoptosis at 24 h, respectively, due to a dramatic increase in oxidative stress [54].

Although many epidemiological studies have been carried out on smokers with lung cancer, there is also evidence to suggest that people living in urban areas have an increased risk of lung cancer due to higher levels of air pollution in these areas. A number of studies have indicated a correlation between lung cancer risk and exposure to urban air pollutants, particularly inhalable and fine particulate matter [55]. In animal experiments, lung toxicity, inflammatory effects, genotoxicity, and rodent carcinogenicity have been demonstrated for diesel exhaust and urban air particulates. In vitro, both can cause oxidative DNA damage, mainly single-strand breaks and 8-oxo-dG (8-oxo-7,8-dihydro-2′-deoxyguanosine). In vivo, even at low-dose levels, diesel exhaust particles can induce oxidative DNA damage in rodent lung tissue [55]. BaP is currently used as the main indicator of PAH levels in air pollution. However, recently, there has been some concern that there may be PAHs with a higher potency of carcinogenicity like dibenz[*a*, *h*]anthracene (DBA) and dibenzo[*a*, *l*]pyrene in air/PAH mixtures that pose even a greater health risk to humans [56].

5. Antioxidants and detoxification

Inside the cell, the harmful effects of free radicals are balanced by the antioxidant action of antioxidant enzymes and nonenzymatic antioxidants that help in the process of detoxification.

Metallothioneins (MTs) are small, cysteine-rich proteins that bind heavy metals and participate in an array of protective stress responses. MTs are found in bacteria, plants, invertebrates, and vertebrates. There are four main mammalian MT isoforms (MT-1 to MT-4) with distinct roles in different tissues. Aerobic organisms are susceptible to damage by reactive oxygen species (ROS) and reactive nitrogen species (RNS). MT protects cells from exposure to various free radical species like the hydroxyl, peroxyl, alkoxyl, and superoxide anion radical and the nitric oxide and nitric dioxide radicals, which react readily with sulfhydryl groups. MT is also important for the regulation of zinc levels and the distribution of this metal in the extracellular space. Since zinc cannot pass easily through membranes, zinc-transporting proteins, Zrt-Irt-like protein or zinc iron permease (ZIPs) and zinc transporters (ZnTs), help to facilitate this process. The presence of Zinc(II) within the cell causes an increase in the major zinc-binding protein metallothionein, and it binds to MTs forming a thermodynamically stable complex. MT can be activated by various stimuli including heavy metal ions, cytokines, growth factors, and oxidative stress within the cell. Cells that display high MT production are resistant to heavy metal toxicity by cadmium, whereas cell lines that cannot synthesize MTs are sensitive to the toxic effects of cadmium [57].

Cytosolic glutathione S-transferases (GSTs) are a supergene family of dimeric enzymes that detoxify a number of carcinogens including polycyclic aromatic hydrocarbons which are some of the principal substrates. The enzyme, GSTM1-1, appears to be particularly effective in dealing with certain PAH derivatives, and at least one large epidemiological study has found a highly significant correlation between the absence of GSTM1–1 activity and adenocarcinoma of the lung in smokers [58]. GSTs require the presence of glutathione in order to fulfill their function of conjugating glutathione (GSH) to cytotoxic and genotoxic lipophilic compounds for their removal from the cell. Interestingly, the presence of intracellular zinc appears to boost glutathione levels in certain cell types [59], and, thus, zinc supplementation may be a useful measure for the prevention of lung cancer from tobacco smoke and environmental factors such as heavy metals by boosting both MT and GST activities [60]. Glutathione supplementation may also be helpful.

Vitamin C (ascorbic acid) and vitamin E (DL-α-tocopherol) treatment together has been reported to result in a significant reduction in smoking-related BaP-DNA adducts in women and suggests that antioxidant supplementation may help to mitigate some of the carcinogenic effects of BaP exposure. It is particularly effective in females with the GSTM1 null genotype, whereas males do not seem to benefit from the same treatment [61].

Black tea polyphenols (theaflavins and epigallocatechin gallate) have been observed to suppress cell proliferation and induce apoptosis during BaP-induced lung carcinogenesis in mice. The occurrence of carcinoma in situ was effectively reduced as a result of this treatment [62] (**Figure 2**).

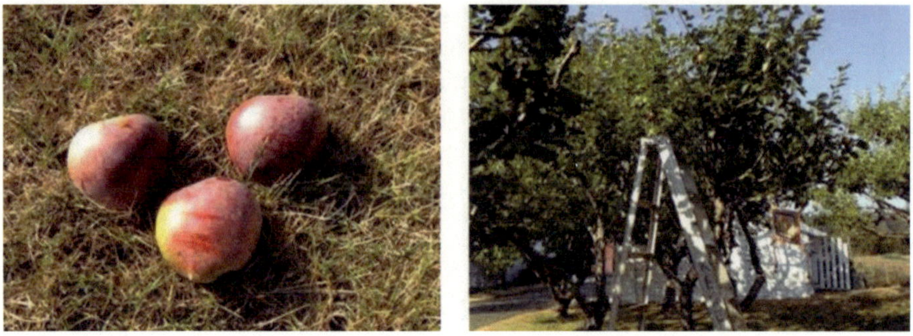

Figure 2.
A crop of BC apples covered with a layer of fine particulate matter from forest fire smoke.

6. Conclusions

Lead and cadmium are two of the heavy metals that are expelled in cigarette smoke. In epidemiological studies, lead and cadmium have been correlated with human cancers including renal and lung, respectively. In animal studies, lead has been found to induce renal tumors in rats and mice, while cadmium inhalation is associated with pulmonary adenocarcinomas in rodents. In addition, oral cadmium in the diet of rats results in tumors of the prostate, testes, and hematopoietic system. Apoptosis or oxidative stress, which can signal cell death, has been observed and reported in cell cultures in response to both metals. As such, these two heavy metals have the potential to cause cancer independently.

The polycyclic aromatic hydrocarbon, benzo(a)pyrene, which is a prominent component of indoor/outdoor air pollution and cigarette smoke, is a well-established carcinogen. BaP-DNA adducts have been observed in lung cancer patients and in experimental animals following BaP exposure. BPDE-DNA adducts have been reported in the white blood cells of occupationally exposed workers and cigarette smokers. There is a strong positive correlation between this type of BaP/BaP metabolite DNA adduct formation and risk for lung cancer in humans. An elevated frequency of BPDE-induced chromosomal aberrations has also been observed in lymphocyte cultures from lung cancer patients. Moreover, animal studies have revealed a highly reproducible association between BaP exposure and respiratory tract tumors in Syrian golden hamsters and lung cancer in mice. BaP treatment of mouse hepatoma cells can cause apoptosis via caspase-3 and caspase-9 activation, mitochondrial dysfunction including a loss in membrane potential and cytosolic release of cytochrome c, and phosphorylation of p53 (Ser15). In a BaP-treated human hepatocellular carcinoma cell line, necrosis is induced at 12 hours and apoptosis at 24 hours, respectively, due to a dramatic increase in oxidative stress. Thus, these results are consistent with a mechanism of carcinogenesis based on an apoptotic model.

Zinc supplementation may be useful for heavy metal detoxification in mammals. Certain antioxidants including vitamin C, vitamin E, black tea polyphenols (theaflavins and epigallocatechin gallate), and flavonoids have been reported to help in mitigating some of the toxic effects of polycyclic aromatic hydrocarbons. Thus, antioxidant supplementation may prove to be an effective measure in reducing the risk of respiratory tract cancers in smokers and from air pollution in developing nations where there is still a significant use of biomass fuels.

In recent years, great progress has been made in banning cigarette smoking from public places around the world due to the proven hazards of secondhand smoke. Some developing nations have also instituted economic and educational programs to discourage the general use of biomass fuels and seasonal burning of paddy fields. Certain countries have legislated stricter laws to deal with irresponsible cigarette smokers, who often start large blazes by discarding their cigarettes and matches outdoors, and, professional arsonists. In places like British Columbia, where there are so many forests and the incidence of forest fires is increasing due to climate change, one extreme solution may be to close public parks during the peak fire season.

Nevertheless, despite these local actions, nothing short of an international effort is required to tackle climate change effectively on a global scale. If countries are to truly cooperate in combatting the rapidly changing conditions on the planet, general goodwill among nations and the cessation of all hostilities embodied in a World Peace Treaty (WPT) seem to be necessary. A ban on the use of nuclear weapons and nuclear testing should also be included in such an agreement since there is already evidence to suggest that atmospheric nuclear explosions have contributed to climate change in addition to greenhouse gases. Economic benefits are likely to be a positive outcome of "green" eco-friendly policies in the long run as awareness about their importance is raised among the general public.

Author details

Chanda Siddoo-Atwal
President and Primary Biochemist of Moondust Cosmetics Ltd, West Vancouver, Canada

*Address all correspondence to: moondustcosmetics@gmail.com

IntechOpen

© 2019 The Author(s). Licensee IntechOpen. This chapter is distributed under the terms of the Creative Commons Attribution License (http://creativecommons.org/licenses/by/3.0), which permits unrestricted use, distribution, and reproduction in any medium, provided the original work is properly cited.

References

[1] Ashraf MW. Levels of heavy metals in popular cigarette brands and exposure to these metals via smoking. The Scientific World Journal. 2012;**2012**:729430. DOI: 10.1100/2012/729430

[2] Chiba M, Masironi R. Toxic and trace elements in tobacco and tobacco smoke. Bulletin of the World Health Organization. 1992;**70**(2):269-275

[3] Caruso RV, O'Connor RJ, Stephens WE, Cummings KM, Fong GT. Toxic metal concentrations in cigarettes obtained from U.S. smokers in 2009: Results from the international tobacco control (ITC) United States Survey Cohort. International Journal of Environmental Research and Public Health. 2014;**11**(1):202-217. DOI: 10.3390/ijerph110100202

[4] Siddoo-Atwal C. Heavy metal carcinogenesis: A possible mechanistic role for apoptosis. Vegetos. 2017;**30**(Special):124. DOI: 10.5958/2229-4473.2017.00046.5

[5] Bruce N, Perez-Padilla R, Albalak R. Indoor air pollution in developing countries: A major environmental and public health challenge. Bulletin of the World Health Organization; Special Theme – Environment and Health. 2000;**78**(9):1078-1092

[6] Eastaugh C. Adaptations of forests to climate change: A multidisciplinary review. IUFRO Occasional Paper No. 21ISSN 1024-414X; 2008

[7] Williams SE. Biodiversity and climate change in the tropical montane rainforests of northern Australia. In: Green RE, Hartley M, Miles L, Scharlemann J, Watson A, Watts O, editors. In: Global Climate Change and Biodiversity. Norwich: Tyndall Center for Climate Change Research; 2003

[8] Hughes L. Climate change and Australia: Trends, projections and impacts. Austral Ecology. 2003;**28**:423-443

[9] Lemmen DS, Warren FJ, editors. Climate Change Impacts and Adaptation. A Canadian Perspective: Natural Resources Canada, Ottawa; 2004

[10] Gillett NP, Weaver AJ, Zwiers FW, Flannigan MD. Detecting the effect of climate change on Canadian forest fires. Geophysical Research Letters. 2004;**31**(18). DOI: 10.1029/2004GL020876

[11] Flannigan MD, Stocks BJ, Wotten BM. Climate change and forest fires. Science of the Total Environment. 2000;**262**:221-229

[12] Adetona O, Reinhardt TE, Domitrovich J, Broyles G, Adetona AM, Kleinman MT, et al. Review of the health effects of wildland fire smoke on wildland firefighters and the public. Inhalation Toxicology. 2016;**28**(3):95-139. DOI: 10.3109/08958378.2016.1145771

[13] McMahon CK, Tsoukalas SN. Polynuclear aromatic hydrocarbons in forest fire smoke. Carcinogenesis. 1978;**3**:61-73

[14] Siddoo-Atwal C. A New Approach to Cancer Risk Assessment: An Overview. LAP Lambert Academic Publishing, OmniScriptum Publishing Group; 2017

[15] Tchounwou PB, Yedjou CG, Patlolla AK, Sutton DJ. Heavy metal toxicity and the environment. Molecular, Clinical, and Environmental Toxicology. 2012;**101**(Experientia Supplementum):133-164

[16] Martin S, Griswold W. Human health effects of heavy metals.

Environmental Science and Technology Briefs for Citizens. 2009;**15**:1-6

[17] International Agency for Research on Cancer (IARC). Overall evaluation of carcinogenicity: An updating of monographs. In: IARC Monographs on the Evaluation of Carcinogenic Risks to Humans. Supplement 7. Volumes 1-42. Lyons, France: IARC; 1987. pp. 230-232

[18] Vijverberg HPM, Oortgiesen M, Leinders T, van Kleef RGDM. Mctal interactions with voltage- and receptor-activated ion channels. Environmental Health Perspectives. 1994;**102**(3):153-158

[19] Goldstein G. Evidence that lead acts as a calcium substitute in second messenger metabolism. Neurotoxicology. 1993;**14**:97-102

[20] Schanne FA, Long GJ, Rosen JF. Lead induced rise in intracellular free calcium is mediated through activation of protein kinase C in osteoblastic bone cells. Biochimica et Biophysica Acta. 1997;**1360**(3):247-254

[21] Simons T. Lead-calcium interactions in cellular lead toxicity. Neurotoxicology. 1993;**14**:77-86

[22] Duchen MR. Contributions of mitochondria to animal physiology: From homeostasis sensor to calcium signalling and cell death. Journal of Physiology. 1999;**516**(1):1-17

[23] Hajnoczky G, Csordas G, Das S, Garcia-Perez C, Saotome M, Sinha Roy S, et al. Mitochondrial calcium signalling and cell death: Approaches for assessing the role of mitochondrial calcium uptake in apoptosis. Cell Calcium. 2006;**40**(5-6):553-560

[24] Martin KR. Targeting apoptosis with dietary bioactive agents. Experimental Biology and Medicine. 2006;**231**:117-129

[25] Sun S, Hail N, Lotan R. Apoptosis as a novel target for cancer chemoprevention. Journal of the National Cancer Institute. 2004;**96**:662-678

[26] Hermes-Lima M, Pereira B, Bechara EJ. Are free radicals involved in lead poisoning? Xenobiotica. 1991;**8**:1085-1090

[27] Erguran-Ilhan I, Cadir B, Koyuncu-Arslan M, Arslan C, Gultcpc FM, Ozkan G. Level of oxidative stress and damage in erythrocytes in apprentices indirectly exposed to lead. Pediatrics International. 2008;**50**(1):45-50

[28] Boffetta P, Fontana L, Stewart P, et al. Occupational exposure to arsenic, cadmium, chromium, lead and nickel, and renal cell carcinoma: A case–control study from Central and Eastern Europe. Occupational and Environmental Medicine. 2011;**68**:723-728

[29] Waalkes MP, Hiwan BA, Ward JM, Devor DE, Goyer RA. Renal tubular tumors and atypical hyperplasias in B6C3F, mice exposed to lead acetate during gestation and lactation occur with minimal chronic nephropathy. Cancer Research. 1995;**55**:5265-5271

[30] Goyer RA. Lead toxicity: Current concerns. Environmental Health Perspectives. 1993;**100**:177-187

[31] Yang JL, Wang LC, Chang CY, Liu TY. Singlet oxygen is the major species participating in the induction of DNA strand breakage and 8-hydrocy-deoxyguanosine adduct by lead acetate. Environmental and Molecular Mutagenesis. 1999;**33**:194-201

[32] Lin RH, Lee CH, Chen WK, Lin-Shiau SY. Studies on cytotoxic and genotoxic effects of cadmium nitrate and lead nitrate in Chinese hamster ovary cells. Environmental and Molecular Mutagenesis. 1994;**23**:143-149

[33] Waalkes MP, Fox DA, States JC, Patierno SR, McCabe MJ. Metals and disorders of cell accumulation: Modulation of apoptosis and cell proliferation. Toxicological Sciences. 2000;**56**:255-261

[34] Waalkes MP, Rehm S. Carcinogenicity of oral cadmium in the male Wistar (WFNCr) rat: Effect of chronic dietary zinc deficiency. Fundamental and Applied Toxicology. 1992;**19**:512

[35] Waalkes MP, Berthan G, editors. Handbook on Metal-Ligand Interactions of Biological Fluids. Vol. 2. New York: Marcel Dekker; 1995. pp. 471-482

[36] Waalkes MP, Misra RR, Chang LW, editors. Toxicology of Metals. Boca Raton, FL: CRC Press; 1996. pp. 231-244

[37] Johri N, Jacquillet G, Unwin R. Heavy metal poisoning: The effects of cadmium on the kidney. BioMetals. 2010;**23**(5):783-792

[38] Harvey RG. Polycyclic Aromatic Hydrocarbons: Chemistry and Carcinogenicity. Cambridge: Cambridge University Press, The Pit Building; 1991

[39] Poster DL, Schantz MM, Sander LC, Wise SA. Analysis of polycyclic aromatic hydrocarbons (PAHs) in environmental samples: A critical review of gas chromatographic (GC) methods. Analytical and Bioanalytical Chemistry. 2006;**386**(4):859-881

[40] Tang D, Santella RM, Balckwood AM, Young TL, Mayer J, Jaretzki A, et al. A molecular epidemiological case-control study of lung cancer. Cancer Epidemiology, Biomarkers & Prevention. 1995;**4**(4):341-346

[41] Shamsuddin AKM, Sinopoli NT, Hemminki K, Boesch RR, Harris CC. Detection of benzo(a)pyrene: DNA adducts in human white blood cells. Cancer Research. 1985;**45**:66-68

[42] Li D, Firozi PF, Wang L-E, Bosken CH, Spitz MR, Hong WK, et al. Sensitivity to DNA damage induced by benzo(*a*)pyrene diol epoxide and risk of lung cancer: A case-control analysis. Cancer Research. 2001;**61**(4):1445-1450

[43] Wei Q, Cheng L, Amos CI, Wang L-E, Guo Z, Hong WK, et al. Repair of tobacco carcinogen-induced DNA adducts and lung cancer risk: A molecular epidemiologic study. Journal of the National Cancer Institute. 2000;**92**(21):1764-1772. DOI: 10.1093/jnci/92.21.1764

[44] Wei Q, Gu J, Cheng L, Bondy ML, Jiang H, Hong WK, et al. Benzo(*a*)pyrene diol epoxide-induced chromosomal aberrations and risk of lung cancer. Cancer Research. 1996;**56**(17):3975-3979

[45] Perera FP, Poirier MC, Yuspa SH, Nakayama J, Jaretzki A, Curnen MM, et al. A pilot project in molecular cancer epidemiology: Determination of benzo[a]pyrene—DNA adducts in animal and human tissues by immunoassays. Carcinogenesis. 1982;**3**(12):1405-1410. DOI: 10.1093/carcin/3.12.1405

[46] Henry MC, Port CD, Bates RR, Kaufman DG. Respiratory tract tumors in hamsters induced by benzo(*a*)pyrene. Cancer Research. 1973;**33**(7):1585-1592

[47] Schreiber H, Saccomanno G, Martin DH, Brennan L. Sequential cytological changes during development of respiratory tract tumors induced in hamsters by benzo(*a*)pyrene-ferric oxide. Cancer Research. 1974;**34**(4):689-698

[48] Kasala ER, Bodduluru LN, Barua CC, Sriram CS, Gogoi R. Benzo(a)pyrene induced lung cancer:

Role of dietary phytochemicals in chemoprevention. Pharmacological Reports. 2015;**67**(5):996-1009. DOI: 10.1016/j.pharep.2015.03.004

[49] Selvendiran K, Banu SM, Sakthisekaran D. Protective effect of piperine on benzo(*a*)pyrene-induced lung carcinogenesis in Swiss albino mice. Clinica Chimica Acta. 2004;**350**(1-2):73-78. DOI: 10.1016/j.cccn.2004.07.004

[50] Kamaraj S, Ramakrishnan G, Anandakumar P, Jagan S, Devaki T. Antioxidant and anticancer efficacy of hesperidin in benzo(a)pyrene induced lung carcinogenesis in mice. Investigational New Drugs. 2009;**27**(3):214-222

[51] Nagahara A, Benjamin H, Storkson J, Krewson J, Sheng K, Liu W, et al. Inhibition of benzo[*a*]pyrene-induced mouse forestomach neoplasia by a principal flavor component of Japanese-style fermented soy sauce. Cancer Research. 1992;**52**(7):1754-1756

[52] Lei W, Yu R, Mandlekar S, Kong A-NT. Induction of apoptosis and activation of interleukin 1β-converting enzyme/Ced-3 protease (Caspase-3) and c-Jun NH_2-terminal kinase 1 by benzo(*a*)pyrene. Cancer Research: Biochemistry and Biophysics. 1998;**58**(10):2102-2106

[53] Ko C-B, Kim S-J, Park C, et al. Benzo(a)pyrene-induced apoptotic death of mouse hepatoma Hepa1c1c7 cells via activation of intrinsic caspase cascade and mitochondrial dysfunction. Toxicology. 1999;**199**(1):35-46. DOI: 10.1016/j.tox.2004.01.039

[54] Jiang Y, Zhou X, Chen X, Yang G, Wang Q, Rao K, et al. Benzo(a)pyrene-induced mitochondrial dysfunction and cell death in p53-null Hep3B cells. Mutation Research. 2011;**26**(1):75-83

[55] Vineis P, Husgafvel-Pursiainen K. Air pollution and cancer: Biomarker studies in human populations. Carcinogenesis. 2005;**26**(11):1846-1855. DOI: 10.1093/carcin/bgi216

[56] Okona-Mensah KB, Battershill J, Boobis A, Fielder R. An approach to investigating the importance of high potency polycyclic aromatic hydrocarbons (PAHs) in the induction of lung cancer by air pollution. Food and Chemical Toxicology. 2005;**43**(7):1103-1116. DOI: 10.1016/j.fct.2005.03.001

[57] Ruttkay-Nedecky B, Nejdl L, Gumulrc J, Zitka O, Masarik M, Eckschlager T, et al. The role of metallothionein in oxidative stress. International Journal of Molecular Sciences. 2013;**14**(3):6044-6066

[58] Ketterer B, Harris JM, Talaska G, Meyer DJ, Pemble SE, Taylor JB, et al. The human glutathione S-transferase supergene family, its polymorphism, and its effects on susceptibility to lung cancer. Environmental Health Perspectives. 1992;**98**:87-94. DOI: 10.1289/ehp.929887

[59] Seagrave J, Tobey RA, Hildebrand CE. Zinc effects on glutathione metabolism relationship to zinc-induced protection from alkylating agents. Biochemical Pharmacology. 1983;**32**(20):3017-3021

[60] Siddoo-Atwal C. Chapter 17: Biological effects of uranium and its decay products on soil microbes, plants, and human. In: Varma A, Tripathi S, Prasad R, editors. Plant Microbe Interface. Cham, Switzerland: Springer; 2019

[61] Mooney LA, Madsen AM, Tang D, Orjuela MA, Tsai W-Y, Garduno ER, et al. Antioxidant vitamin supplementation reduces benzo(*a*)pyrene-DNA adducts and

potential cancer risk in female smokers. Cancer Epidemiology, Biomarkers & Prevention. 2005;**14**(1):237-242

[62] Banerjee S, Manna S, Saha P, Panda C, Das S. Black tea polyphenols suppress cell proliferation and induce apoptosis during benzo(a) pyrene-induced lung carcinogenesis. European Journal of Cancer Prevention. 2005;**14**(3):215-221

Section 2

Health Risks, Toxicological and Cellular Tissue Effects of Heavy Metals

Chapter 4

Mercury Toxicity in Public Health

Narjala Rama Jyothi
and Nainar Abdulkhader Mohamed Farook

Abstract

Mercury was the name of the Roman messenger of god who can move really fast. It is also called as quicksilver due to its fast movement and silvery tinge. Liquid metal state mercury (Hg) has little to no solubility and is not poisonous. But the liquid mercury can vaporize, and gaseous mercury becomes poisonous due to its nature of being absorbed into the blood. Mercury in +2 state is more poisonous due to high solubility. Mercury is the only metal that exists in liquid state at normal temperature and pressure. Mercury poisoning occurs by exposure to mercury, i.e., acute and chronic exposures. Symptoms of mercury poisoning depend on the type, dose, method, and duration of exposure. Mercury poisoning effects on the human body are not limited to reddishness of hands and feet; renal failures; cardiovascular, liver, brain, and hormonal issues; and intestinal ulceration. The present chapter describes the mercury sources, types of exposures, types of poisoning, treatments, and preventive measures of mercury poisoning.

Keywords: mercury, heavy metal toxicity, sources, exposure of mercury, mercury poisoning, toxicity of mercury, prevention mercury toxicity

1. Introduction

Heavy metal contamination is a serious problem to the environment, because they are not only biodegradable but also toxic to living organisms. The metals such as cadmium, mercury, and lead are owing much more interest to environmental scientists due to their accumulation in vital organs of the living beings. Once these metals are absorbed into the human body, they can be a threat with more health issues [1]. The absorbed mercury in humans becomes more toxic due to its prolonged half-life and lack of decomposition, and its interaction is not limited with various enzymes and proteins. Mercury has a great affinity with thiol group in proteins and causes many diseases.

Mercury is the only metal that exists in liquid state among the total periodic table elements. It is very important to measure the concentration of mercury in the environment due to its bioaccumulative property in its elemental and organic forms (i.e., methylmercury) and toxic nature. Mercury (Hg) is a naturally occurring element that is toxic in nature. According to the US Environmental Protection Agency, the safe limit of mercury ion in drinking water is 10 nM to avoid the serious health problems to humans [2]. Mercury is a pollutant of global concern. The Minamata Convention on Mercury entered into force from 2017, regarding the protection of human and environmental health. A recent review reported about the worldwide

IntechOpen

and regional time trends in total mercury levels in the human blood and breast milk and their associations with health effects [3].

Mercury is a metal that appears as silver balls, and its liquid form is called elemental mercury. Mercury in the environment can exist in different forms, such as mercurous ion (Hg^{+1}), mercuric ion (Hg^{+2}), methylmercury (CH_3Hg^+), ethylmercury ($C_2H_5Hg^+$), and phenylmercury ($C_6H_5Hg^+$). The chemical forms of mercury in the environment are broadly divided into three, i.e., (1) elemental mercury, (2) inorganic salts, and (3) organic compounds.

Elemental mercury: The atmosphere consists of mercury in elemental form, and at room temperature it is present in liquid form. It is used in thermometers and fluorescent bulbs.

Inorganic mercury: It occurs in several forms: metallic (Hg), mercurous (Hg^{1+}), or mercuric form (Hg^{2+}). This is present in crystal form, and it is used in pesticides and antiseptics.

Organic mercury: It is in the forms of aryl and alkyl. Methylmercury is the best example; it mixes with the food chain.

Nagpal et al. [4] reviewed the mercury exposure and health effects of dental personnel. Bernhoft [5] reviewed about the mercury toxicity and its treatments. Driscoll et al. [6] reviewed the sources, pathways, and effects of mercury in global environment. O'Connor et al. [7] reviewed about the mercury speciation, transformation, and transportation in soils, atmospheric flux, and implications for risk management. Taber et al. [8] studied the mercury exposure and effects across the life span. Antoszczyszyn and Michalska [9] reported the potential risk of environmental contamination by mercury contained in Polish coal mining waste. The toxic effects of mercury on human beings depend on several factors, such as chemical form of mercury, age, health condition of person exposed, and type of exposure. A study [10] regarding mercury toxicity reported that yearly around 60,000 babies were born with neurological problems due to their mothers poisoned with mercury.

The present chapter describes the mercury sources, types of exposures, types of poisoning, and preventions to avoid mercury poisoning.

2. Sources of mercury

The sources of mercury in the environment are classified into two types, i.e., natural and anthropogenic. The natural and anthropogenic sources of mercury in the environment are presented in **Table 1**.

Sources of mercury	
Natural	**Anthropogenic**
1. Volcanoes	1. Hydroelectric
2. Forest fires	2. Mining
3. Cinnabar (ore)	3. Pulp industry
4. Fossil fuel (coal and petroleum)	4. Paper industry
	5. Medical waste
	6. Municipal waste
	7. Coal using power plant

Table 1.
Sources of mercury.

3. Natural sources

A number of studies worldwide reported the determination of mercury in naturally available sources, such as volcanic eruptions, forest fires, cinnabar, and fossil fuels.

Regarding volcanic eruptions, a research study reported the determination of mercury at Masaya caldera complex, Santiago, Nicaragua. This study found the concentration of mercury at 232 selected points at the research area. They found higher concentrations of Hg(0) at their sampling sites [11]. Speciation of mercury in volcanic eruptions at Mount Etna, Sicily, Italy, was reported by Baganto et al. [12]. This study represents a systematic characterization of mercury partitioning between gaseous mercury and particulate forms in the volcanic eruptions.

Another study reported the determination of mercury in the volcanic eruptions at Kilauea volcano, Hawaii. This study found the low concentrations of mercury at soils with more sulfur content [13]. In Western Wyoming, Hg accumulation was examined between burned and unburned sampling sites with the total tree species composition. Results show that Hg emitted from forest fires depends on the forest fire intensity and Hg formation before the firing [14]. Atmospheric mercury species emitted due to forest fires were studied in three rural sites (southern Quebec, Canada, and northern New York). MODIS satellite reports show forest fires transmitted from Quebec, Canada to northern New York. Accumulation of Hg species in the atmosphere after the forest fire incidents is higher than the normal environmental conditions [15]. In Europe and North African countries, mercury emissions from forest fires are studied based on ground data and phytomass [16].

Mercury is a volatile metal due to its nature; it easily gets away from its deposits and enters into the atmosphere. Globally it was reported that 2000 to 8000 metric tons of Hg emissions takes place during the years 1550–1880. In Florida and the USA, speciation of mercury emissions was studied. Globally more Hg emissions are happening in industrialized areas [17]. At present years, industrial areas are the interesting research zones due to its huge Hg emissions; transport modeling is the tool used for calculating Hg emissions, and this is used for the analysis of Hg emissions in industrial zones [18].

Cinnabar is a toxic mercury sulfide (HgS), and it is the main ore of mercury. It is chemically inert and has low toxic potential when taken orally. Isonzo river (Gulf of Trieste) is the area in which high cinnabar is accumulated and Hg is bounded to it as fine particles [19]. Liu et al. [20] reported that Hg is a toxic metal. Cinnabar is used in Chinese medicines. Heating the ore leads to production of vapors, which are dangerous if inhaled and enter the stomach where it is not absorbed and finally deposits on the kidneys. Prolonged use of cinnabar inhalation leads to kidney damage.

There are two fish species, namely, piscivorous (northern pike and walleye) and non-piscivorous (lake white fish and longnose sucker). Hg concentration depends on fish species and type of reservoirs. After 5 years of rapid filling of reservoirs with water, the Hg level increases, and later in 10 years, Hg concentration will decrease [21]. Hydroelectric reservoirs are increasing rapidly due to the need of electricity. The present studies reported the Hg accumulation in water before and after flooding. The conversion of Hg to MeHg in the environment leads to an increase in the toxicity in water. In order to decline the toxicity, intensive fishing is the best remedy. Adding selenium to water is another best method to decrease the Hg content in water. MeHg is deposited in fishes, and eating such type of fishes leads to severe health risks [22]. Bodaly et al. [23] conducted a study on fish in the boreal reservoir of Northern Manitoba, Canada. In lake white fish, the Hg concentration after floods as post-impoundment is 0.2–0.4 $\mu g\ g^{-1}$ and pre-impoundment is 0.06–0.14 $\mu g\ g^{-1}$. Hg concentration in northern spike and walleye after flooding as below post-impoundment is 0.7–2.6 $\mu g\ g^{-1}$ and pre-impoundment is 0.19–0.047 $\mu g\ g^{-1}$.

Insect larvae are another source of storage of Hg and MeHg in hydroelectric reservoir. The storage of mercury in hydroelectric reservoir is higher than natural lakes. The flooded soil is one of major sources for insect larvae which is studied by Tremblay and Lucotte [24]. Mining is the major anthropogenic source for the release of tones of mercury into the environment. In global consideration Brazil is the topmost country in gold production; nearly 2000 tons of mercury was released into the environment. In some areas there is a lot of Hg accumulation taking place without gold mining; it is due to man-made mistakes (sediments, human hair, and urine) [25].

Appleton et al. [26] reported that Naboc River water is highly contaminated with Hg. Rice paddy fields are present in the Naboc area and were irrigated with Naboc River water, so the soil was highly contaminated with mercury. In contrast the corn and banana crops that are not irrigated with Naboc river water produced mercury-free crops.

Amalgamation is the process of using the mercury in mining gold and silver. Patio process is used in Spanish colonial America, Australia, Southeast Asia, and England. From 1550 to 1930, 260,000 tons of mercury was released into the atmosphere. South America (Amazon), China, Southeast Asia, and African countries have been using widely mercury amalgamation. Mining is the major anthropogenic source; 10% of mercury emissions is involved due to this. About 300 tons of mercury is released into the environment through gold and silver mining since the last 500 years [27].

Malm et al. [28] performed research studies on the sediments of Madeira River basin. The sediment particles are amalgamated with mercury; 30% of mercury was released into the river water, whereas 20% of mercury was released into the atmosphere.

4. Types of exposure

Mercury exposure to the humans can take place in three ways, through dermal contact from soil, through drinking water, and through inhalation of the atmosphere and intake by food. The mercury in the atmosphere can be dissolved into water and can change into a more toxic form of methylmercury by micro-organisms. Methylmercury is more toxic than elemental mercury. The historical incident of Minamata, Japan, was an evidence of the bioaccumulation of methylmercury in fishes in which it can enter into the food web and finally to the humans. The levels of methylmercury in fish depend on what they eat, how long they live, and how high they are in food chain.

There are two types of exposures that we can observe in human populations with mercury, i.e., acute exposure and chronic exposure. Acute exposure to inorganic mercury or mercuric salts is mostly like through oral route. Chronic exposure is usually related to prolonged exposure during occupational incidents.

The exposure of mercury has been historically reported since a few hundreds of years. Inorganic mercury compounds were used in skin ointments which were used to treat some skin diseases in ancient Egypt. In Korea, occupational mercury exposure to humans was observed in fluorescent lamp manufacturing and silver refining plants. In normal populations, mercury exposure is through inhalation by burning charms [29].

Based on the literature, it is concluded that there are no significant toxicological effects observed by the ingestion of elemental mercury by a healthy person because of its poor absorbance into the gastrointestinal tract. The chronic exposure to the mercury vapor mostly affects the central nervous system and the kidneys. The major exposure by the human population to the mercury vapor is through inhalation route, because 80% of the mercury can reach the lungs and be dissolved in the blood reaching the different organs [30].

5. Types of poisoning

Mercury is a toxic metal, and it occurs naturally and exists in elemental (or metallic), inorganic (mercuric chloride), and organic (methyl- and ethylmercury) forms. Thiomersal (sodium ethylmercury thiosalicylate) contains 49.6% ethylmercury. It is used as a preservative in children vaccines. According to According to American Academy of Pediatricians (AAP) the vaccinated children are pronging to Autism due to Hg present in Thiomersal [31].

Clarkson et al. [32] reported that the Hg poisoning results in psychiatric disturbances due to CNS dysfunction and it also effects listening and speaking abnormalities. Intention tremor is the abnormality created in speech and mouth disorders [33].

Sensory motor problems and defects (touch, excessive mouthing) are caused by mercury toxicity. According to a study [34], ADHD and ASD are the few abnormalities related to mental retardation, and abnormal behavior is exhibited by the affected people. Some of the abnormal behaviors [35] are seen due to mercury toxic nature, i.e., there is no controlled-on mind activities in babies. Mercury poisoning also affects the memory and involuntary actions.

Mercury toxicology effects on the visions of children and adults include poor visibility, blurriness, and no fixed visuality. Mercury toxic nature not only affects mental health, but also it creates several physical disturbances, such as hyper−/hypotonia [36]. Muscle weakness, shivering in arm, and few disturbances will occur in some patients, and in few cases, the complete chance of paralysis is also studied [37].

Poor blood circulation led to a change in color of feet and hands to red and blue color which is one of the toxic effects of mercury poisoning [38]. Sweating-related problems, i.e., excessive sweating (acrodynia) and fast heartbeat, are seen in few adults [39].

The toxic nature of mercury mostly effects gastrointestinal systems of humans. The inhalation of mercury led to several discomforts in the abdominal region such as gut-related problems, lesions in colon, and severe abdominal pain [40].

The historical incident happened regarding mercury compound poisoning in Minamata Bay, Japan, in 1956. The important features of Minamata diseases are discussed here under.

6. Minamata disease

It is a chronic disease due to methylmercury coming from industrial wastes, and such wastes deposit in water sources as sediments. The deposited methylmercury enters the fishes available in the water sources and enters the food chain and finally reaches the humans. In New Mexico, USA, research were performed on seed grain treated with methylmercury and reported that those grains are exposed to Minamata disease (https://www.medicinenet.com/script/main/art.asp? articlekey=14084). Akagi et al. [41] reported the methylmercury dose based on umbilical cord concentrations of the patients suffering from Minamata disease.

Matsumoto et al. [42] had reported the clinical survey regarding Minamata disease in children and found symptoms such as cerebral palsy. Ekino et al. [43] studied methylmercury poisoning effects and reviewed the history of its toxicity (1950–1968) for about 20 years and found that methylmercury spread from Minamata Bay to Shiranui Sea.

The consumption of fish or shellfish with mercury by pregnant women affects the fetus brain (Harada 1978). Another study [44] reported at Minamata disease affected people in Kumamoto and found the damage of cerebral cortex.

In addition to the Minamata disease, the other major disease caused due to the mercury poisoning through teething powder is pink disease, in which the foot and hand turn into pink color. The pink disease-affected children were found to have high mercury content in their urine samples [45]. Other than the teething powder, the reasons for the pink disease in young children were viral infections and nutrition deficiency [46].

7. Renal and bone-related effects due to mercury poisoning

Gottelli et al. [47] have studied the effect of mercury on renal function. Phenylmercury enters in the renal tubes through the contaminated diapers, with the excretion of gamma glutamyl transpeptidase in renal cells leading to increase urinary volume and toxicity. Osteoporosis and osteopenia diseases in Korean men due to mercury were studied by Kim et al. [48]. The analysis was performed on Korean men's blood samples, and high mercury range in younger people was found. The analysis was performed on different categories people like alcoholic and in fish consumers, the content of mercury range was found in them due to their intakes. Parejo et al. [49] have studied some cases related to low bone density which is due to the contaminated food and water sources. The intake of Hg was calculated in women in Spain, and studies were related on bone disorder reasons. Garcia et al. [50] reveal that bone disorders, like osteoporosis, are due to heavy toxic metals like mercury, etc. and due to dietary mercury intake which is the reason of accumulation of mercury in the bones. In a study of 158 women, 25.29 μg/day of dietary heavy metal intake leads to several osteoporosis cases and fracturing. Dainowski et al. [51] studied the total mercury (THg) concentration on muscle, kidney, and liver of red foxes in Western Alaska. It was seen that total mercury concentration in hair is correlated with muscle, kidney, and liver. The major reason of mercury content is due to industrialization in Arctic areas. Accumulation of mercury in human tissues and severe knee-related problems were studied by Bogacka et al. [52]. In northwestern Poland, the total mercury percentage in women cartilage was high compared to selenium, and moreover knee joint-related problems in patients are also due to selenium to total mercury ratio.

8. Hormonal effects of mercury poisoning

Adipogenesis is the process of cell differentiation and study on adipocytes (lipocytes, fat cells). Adiposeness is the process of study modules of cell differentiation. Telapolu et al. [53] studied on MD-1, it is a polyherbal used in management of Diabetes mellitus. α-Glycosidase and α-amylase are the two carbohydrate digestive enzymes, HAEF is the extract, and its effect on digestive enzymes was studied. The effect of MD-1 on adipogenesis was studied, and the effect of HAEF on mRNA expression of peroxisome proliferator-activated receptor gamma (PPARγ) and glucose transporter 4 (GLUT4) in 3T3L1 adipocytes was investigated.

9. Liver-related effects due to mercury poisoning

Hussain et al. [54] studied about the effects of mercurous chloride on the liver, brain, and kidney which are due to enzymes like superoxide dismutase (SOD), glutathione peroxidase (GPx), and glutathione reductase. The increase in the mercury levels is correlated with enzyme activities, and generation of reactive oxygen species (ROS) is the cause of mercury accumulation. Fish is the major source of mercury; consuming such mercury stored in fish leads to exposure of human tissues to high mercury levels. Pelletier et al. [55] examined by checking mercury levels in rodents as they are exposed frequently with *Rhododendron tomentosum* extract and their blood is with higher mercury levels. Williams et al. [56] reported flurbiprofen (anti-inflammatory drug) is the cause of bone resorption disease. Cyclooxygenase inhibitor is the cause of periodontal disease in beagles.

Crespo et al. [57] studied *Lactobacillus casei effect on mercury*, and results show the decreased methylmercury bioavailability in acutely exposed mice. Mercury accumulation in the liver and kidney was not affected by *Lactobacillus* supplementation. Adult male rats are exposed to Labrador tea and antibiotic cocktail in which methylmercury is present in it. It was observed that when the rats were treated with antibiotics, increased Hg levels in blood levels were observed. El- Demerdash [58] studies reported on oxidative stress of Hg and selenium. Rats were given Hg (0.5 μmol/ml), for 5 days, and several biochemical assays were done on them, and it was observed that after the Hg treatment, the protein content in the brain and liver was decreased.

10. Prevention measures of mercury poisoning

Consuming of fish two servings per a week leads to good cordial health, but the presence of mercury, especially in oil fish like salmon and sardines, leads to an increased risk of cardiovascular health. Avoiding such sort of fish is one of the best prevention measures. Davis (http://www.emedicine health.com/mercury_poisoning/article_em.htm) reported on the prevention measures of mercury at various areas. In home broken thermometers and fluorescent light tubes are the major sources; awareness and preventive measures should be taken into account in disposing them far away. Dental amalgam fillings should be avoided by mercury, and any other alternative material should be used. The mothers feeding the infants should be most aware of taking fishes because the mercury content present may affect the infant brain and spine; this is one of the good preventive measures. Thiomersal is the preservative used in flu vaccines; usage of such vaccines may affect the child, so clear precautions are needed for preventing mercury entry into children through the vaccine.

Author details

Narjala Rama Jyothi[1*] and Nainar Abdulkhader Mohamed Farook[2]

1 Department of Chemistry, School of Engineering, Sri Padmavathi Mahila Visvavidyalayam, Tirupati, Andhra Pradesh, India

2 Department of Chemistry, Khadir Mohideen College, Adhirampattinam, Tamil Nadu, India

*Address all correspondence to: ramadasaradhi@gmail.com

IntechOpen

© 2020 The Author(s). Licensee IntechOpen. This chapter is distributed under the terms of the Creative Commons Attribution License (http://creativecommons.org/licenses/by/3.0), which permits unrestricted use, distribution, and reproduction in any medium, provided the original work is properly cited.

References

[1] Xie YL, Zhao SQ, Ye HL, Yuan J, Song P, Hu SQ. Graphene/CeO_2 hybrid materials for the simultaneous electrochemical detection of cadmium (II), copper(II), and mercury(II). Journal of Electroanalytical Chemistry. 2015;**757**:235-242

[2] USEPA. United States Environmental Protection Agency, National Primary Drinking Water Regulations. 2009. Available from: http://www.epa.gov

[3] Sharma BM, Sanka O, Kalina J, Scheringer M. An overview of worldwide and regional time trends in total mercury levels in human blood and breast milk from 1966 to 2015 and their associations with health effects. Environmental International. 2019;**125**:300-319

[4] Nagpal N, Bettiol SS, Isham A, Hoang H, Crocombe LA. A review of mercury exposure and health of dental personnel. Safety and Health at Work. 2017;**8**:1-10

[5] Bernhoft RA. Mercury toxicity and treatment: A review of the literature. Journal of Environmental and Public Health. 2012;**2012**: Article ID: 460508

[6] Driscoll CT, Mason RP, Chan HM, Jacob DJ, Pirrone N. Mercury as a global pollutant: Sources, pathways, and effects. Environmental Science and Technology. 2013;**47**:4967-4983

[7] O'Connor D, Hou D, Ok YS, Mulder J, Duan L, Wu Q, et al. Mercury speciation, transportation, and transportation in soils, atmospheric flux and implications for risk management: A critical review. Environmental International. 2019;**126**:747-761

[8] Taber KH, Hurley RA. Mercury exposure: Effects across the lifespan. The Journal of Neuropsychiatry and Clinical Neurosciences. 2008;**20**(4):384-389

[9] Antoszczyszyn T, Michalska A. The potential risk of environmental contamination by mercury contained in polish coal mining waste. Journal of Sustainable Mining. 2016;**15**:191-196

[10] Schrope M. US to take temperature of mercury threat. Nature. 2001;**409**:124

[11] Crenshaw WB, Williams SN, Stoiber RE. Fault location by radon and mercury detection at an active volcano in Nicaragua. Nature. 1982;**300**:345-346

[12] Baganto E, Aiuppa A, Parello F, Calabrese S, Alessandro WD, Mather TA, et al. Degassing of gaseous (elemental and reactive) and particulate mercury from Mount Etna volcano (southern Italy). Atmospheric Environment. 2007;**41**(35):7377-7388

[13] Cox ME. Summit out gassing as indicated by radon mercury and pH mapping, Kilauea volcano, Hawaii. Journal of Volcanology and Geothermal Research. 1983;**16**(1-2):131-151

[14] Biswas A, Blum JD, Klaue B, Keeler GJ. Release of mercury form rocky mountain forest fires. Global Biogeochemical Cycles. 2007;**21**:GB1002

[15] Wang Y, Huang J, Zananski TJ, Hopke PK, Holsen TM. Impacts of the Canadian forest fires on atmospheric mercury and carbonaceous particles in northern New York. Environmental Science and Technology. 2010;**44**(22):8435-8440

[16] Cinnirella S, Pirrone N. Spatial and temporal distributions of mercury emissions form forest fires in Mediterranean region and Russian federation. Atmospheric Environment. 2006;**40**(38):7346-7361

[17] Hanisch C. Where is mercury deposition coming from? Environmental Science and Technology. 1998;**3297**:176A-179A

[18] Pacyna JM, Munch J. Anthropogenic mercury emission in Europe. Water, Air, and Soil Pollution. 1991;**56**(1):51-61

[19] Covelli S, Faganeli J, Horvat M, Brambati A. Mercury contamination of coastal sediments as the results of long-term cinnabar mining activity (Gulf of Trieste, northern Adriatic Sea). Applied Geochemistry. 2001;**16**(50):541-558

[20] Liu J, Shi JZ, Yu LM, Goyer RA, Waalkes MP. Mercury in traditional medicines: Is cinnabar toxicologically similar to common mercurials? Experimental Biology and Medicine. 2008;**233**(7):810-817

[21] Verdon R, Brouard D, Demers C, Lalumiere R, Laperle M, Schetagne R. Mercury evolution (1978-1988) in fishes of the La Grande hydroelectric complex, Quebec, Canada. Water, Air, and Soil Pollution. 1991;**56**(1):405-417

[22] Maliman M, Stepnuk L, Cicek N, Bodaly RAD. Strategies to lower methyl mercury concentrations in hydroelectric reservoirs and lakes: A review. The Science of the Total Environment. 2006;**368**(1):224-235

[23] Bodaly RA, Jansen WA, Majewski AR, Fudge JP, Strange NE, Derksen AJ, et al. Postimpoundment time course of increased mercury concentrations in fish in hydroelectric reservoirs of northern Manitoba, Canada. Archives of Environmental Contamination and Toxicology. 2007;**53**(3):379-389

[24] Tremblay A, Lucotte M. Accumulation of total mercury and methyl mercury in insect larvae of hydroelectric reservoirs. Canadian Journal of Fisheries and Aquatic Sciences. 1997;**54**(4):832-841

[25] Malm O. Gold mining as a source of mercury exposure in the Brazilian Amazon. Environmental Research. 1998;**77**(2):73-78

[26] Appleton JD, Weeks JM, Calvez JPS, Beinhoff C. Impacts of mercury contaminated mining waste on soil quality, crops, bivalves, and fish in the Naboc river area, Mindanao, Philippines. Science of the Total Environment. 2006;**354**(2-3):198-211

[27] Lacerda LD. Global mercury emissions from gold and silver mining. Water, Air, and Soil Pollution. 1997;**97**(3-4):209-221

[28] Malm O, Pfeiffer WC, Souza CMM, Reuther R. Mercury pollution due to gold mining in the Madeira river basin, Brazil. Ambio. 1990;**19**(1):11-15

[29] Lee HY, Kang GH, Nam KH, Kim MH, Jung BH, Kang HD, et al. Acute mercury vapor inhalation toxicity after burning charms: A case report. Korean Journal of Critical Care Medicine. 2010;**25**(3):182-185. (Korean)

[30] Kim MK, Zoh KD. Fate and transport of mercury in environmental media and human exposure. Journal of Preventive Medicine and Public Health. 2012;**45**:335-343

[31] Bernard S, Enayati A, Redwood L, Roger H, Binstock T. Autism: A Unique Form of Mercury Poisoning. 2000. Available from: http://citeseerx.ist.psu.edu/viewdoc/download?doi=10.1.1.384.1456& rep=rep1 &type=pdf

[32] Clarkson T. The toxicology of mercury. Critical Reviews in Clinical Laboratory Sciences. 1997;**34**(3):369-403

[33] Kark RA, Poskanzer DC, Bullock JD, Boylen G. Mercury poisoning and its treatment with N-acetyl-D,

L-penicillamine. New England Journal of Medicine. 1971;**285**(1):10-16

[34] Gillberg C, Coleman M. The Biology of the Autistic Syndromes. 2nd ed. London, UK; Mac Keith Press; 1992

[35] Teitelbaum P, Teitelbaum O, Nye J, Fryman J, Maurer RG. Movement analysis in infancy may be useful for early diagnosis of autism. Proceedings of theNational Academy of Sciences, USA. 1998;**75**:13982-13987

[36] Nordin V, Gillberg C. Autism Spectrum disorders in children with physical or mental disability or both. I: Clinical and epidemiological aspects. Developmental Medicine and Child Neurology. 1996;**8**(4):297-313

[37] Amin-Zaki L, Majeed MA, Clarkson TW, Greenwood MR. Methylmercury poisoning in Iraqi children: Clinical observations over two years. British Medical Journal. 1978;**1**:613-616

[38] Carpenter PK, Morris D. Association of acrocyanosis with Asperger's syndrome. Journal of Mental Deficiency Research. 1990;**34**:87-90

[39] Farnsworth D. Pink Disease Survey Results. Pink Disease Support Group Site. 1997. Available from: www.users.bigpond.com/difarnsworth

[40] Horvath K, Papadimitriou JC, Rabsztyn A, Drachenberg C, Tildon JT. Gastrointestinalabnormalitiesinchildren with autistic disorder. Journal of Pediatrics. 1999;**135**(5):559-563

[41] Akagi H, Grandjean P, Takizawa Y, Weihe P. Methyl mercury dose estimation from umbilical cord concentrations in patients with Minamata disease. Environmental Research. 1998;**77**:98-103

[42] Matsumoto H, Koya G, Takeuchi T. Fetal Minamata disease: A neuropathological study of two cases of intrauterine intoxication by a methylmercury compound. Journal of Neuropathology and Experimental Neurology. 1965;**24**(4):563-574

[43] Ekino S, Susa M, Ninomiya T, Imamura K, Kitamura T. Minamata disease revisited: An update on the acute and chronic manifestations of methyl mercury poisoning. Journal of Neurological Sciences. 2007;**262**(1-2):131-144

[44] Eto K. Review article: Pathology of Minamata disease. Toxicologic Pathology. 1997;**25**(6):614-623

[45] Dinehart SM, Dillard R, Raimer SS, Cobos R, Pupo R. Cutaneous manifestations of Acrodynia (pink disease). Archives of Dermatology. 1988;**124**(1):107-109

[46] Dally A. The rise and fall of pink disease. Social History of Medicine. 1997;**10**(2):291-304

[47] Gotelli CA, Astolfi E, Cox C, Cernichiari E, Clarkson TW. Early biochemical effects of an organic mercury fungicide on infants: "dose makes the poison". Science. 1985;**227**(4687):638-640

[48] Kim YH, Shim JY, Seo MS, Yim HJ, Cho MR. Relationship between blood mercury concentration and bone mineral density in Korean men in the 2008-2010 Korean national health nutrition examination survey. Korean Journal of Family Medicine. 2016;**37**(5):273-278

[49] Parejo LMP, Aliga I, Macias MLC, Hernandez OL, Martin RR, Martin SR, et al. Evaluation of the dietary intake of cadmium, lead and mercury and its relationship with bone health among postmenopausal women in Spain. International Journal of Environmental Research and Public Health. 2017;**14**(6):564

[50] Garcia JML, Parejo LMP, Martin RR, Moran JM, Zamorano JDP, Aliaga IJ,

et al. Dietary intake of cadmium, lead and mercury and its association with bone health in healthy premenopausal women. Journal of Environmental Research and Public Health. 2017;**14**(12):1437

[51] Dainowski BH, Duffy LK, Mcintyre J, Jones P. Hair and bone as predictors of tissular mercury concentrations in the Western Alaska red fox, *Vulpes vulpes*. The Science of the Total Environment. 2015;**518-519**:526-533

[52] Bogacka DIK, Arendarczyk NL, Kot K, Ciosek Z, Zietek P, Karaczun M, et al. Effects of biological factors and health condition on mercury and selenium concentrations in the cartilage, meniscus and anterior cruciate ligament. Journal of Trace Elements in Medicine and Biology. 2017;**44**:201-208

[53] Telapolu S, Kalachavedu M, Punnoose AM, Bilikere D. MD-1, a poly herbal formulation indicated in diabetes mellitus ameliorates glucose uptake and inhibits adipogenisis-an in vitro study. BMC Complementary and Alternative Medicine. 2018;**18**:113

[54] Hussain S, Atkinson A, Thompson SJ, Khan AT. Accumulation of mercury and its effects on antioxidant enzymes in brain, liver, and kidneys of mice. Journal of Environmental Science and Health, Part B. 1999;**34**:645-660

[55] Pelletier G, Feng YL, Leingartner K, Black P. Co-administration of *Rhododendron tomentosum* extract does not affect mercury tissue concentrations and excretion rate in methylmercury-treated adult male rats. BMC Research Notes. 2019;**12**: Article Number 369

[56] Williams RC, Jeffcoat MK, Kaplan ML, Goldhaber P, Johnson HG, Wechter WJ. Flurbiprofen: A potent inhibitor of alveolar bone resorption in beagles. Science. 1985;**227**(4687): 640-642

[57] Jadán-Piedra C, Crespo Á, Monedero V, Vélez D, Devesa V, Zúñiga M. Effect of lactic acid bacterial on mercury toxicokinetic. Food and Chemical Toxicology. 2019;**128**:147-153

[58] El-Demerdash FM. Effects of selenium and mercury on the enzymatic activities and lipid peroxidation in brain, liver, and blood of rats. Journal of Environmental Science and Health Part B. 2001;**36**(4):488-499

Chapter 5

Health Risks of Potentially Toxic Metals Contaminated Water

Om Prakash Bansal

Abstract

Groundwater which fulfills globally 50–80% need of drinking water, due to Anthropogenic and geologic activities, has been continuously contaminated by potentially toxic metals, causing a range of effects to animals and citizenry. In the developing countries, about 80% of diseases are waterborne diseases. Bio accumulation of these metals in citizenry due to intake of contaminated vegetables, fruits, fishes, seafood and drinking water and beverages causes a serious threat to citizenry. Toxicity of these metals is due to metabolic interference and mutagenesis, interference in the normal functioning of structural proteins, enzymes, and nucleic acids by binding them, adversely affecting the immune and hematopoietic systems in citizenry and animals. The toxic metals also enrich antibiotic resistant microbes particularly bacteria by Co-selection (occurring by Co-resistance and cross-resistance) as it promotes antibiotic resistance in bacteria even in absence of antibiotics. These metals in living cells cause cytotoxicity, oxidative stress resulting in the damages of antioxidants, enzyme inhibition, loss of DNA repair mechanism, protein dysfunction and damage to lipid per oxidase. Endocrine disruption, neuro-developmental toxicity, biosynthesis of hemoglobin, metabolism of vitamin D, renal toxicity, damage to central nervous system, hearing speech and visual disorders, hypertension, anemia, dementia, hematemesis, bladder, lung, nose, larynx, prostate cancer, and bone diseases are some other health's risks to human.

Keywords: pollution, human, potentially toxic metals, health risks, heavy metals resistance, fishes

1. Introduction

Water the "life-blood of the biosphere" may be an alcahest which dissolves different chemicals and environmental pollutants. Globally, groundwater is the main source of domestic drinking water both in rural and urban areas and fulfills approximately 80% need of drinking water in the rural areas and 50% of urban water need. As surface water infiltrates to unconfined aquifers easily, these aquifers are contaminated very easily. The pollution of groundwater causes significant alteration in the environment. The most sources of lakes, rivers, ponds, and streams are the groundwater. When contaminated groundwater is supplied to those sources, the surface water is additionally contaminated which causes harm to birds, animals, and plants. Because of population growth over the last 50 years, the abstraction of groundwater has increased leading to reduce natural discharge flows and groundwater quality. Groundwater quality is additionally suffering from recharge rate and recharge quality. Existence of human on earth without potentially toxic metals is not possible.

These potentially toxic metals (Cd, Cu, Pb, Zn, Cr (III), Cr (VI), and Hg) have high relative atomic mass and density. Hindu Business on Feb 20, 2019 reported that "more than forty million people in rural India drinks to water contaminated by heavy metals, arsenic, fluoride, etc." The results are devastating. Diarrhea, often caused by exposure to fecal matter, kills 600,000 Indians per annum and waterborne diseases throughout the Ganges basin. In India, 25% of water sources is River Ganga. These metals participate within the redox reactions and are an important part of enzymes. Cobalt is a constituent of vitamin B_{12}, and manganese acts as an activator of the enzymes within the physical body [1]. Copper is important for enzyme ascorbate oxidase, cytochrome oxidase, plastocyanin oxidase, and photosynthesis in plants. As these metals cannot be degraded, they persist in the environment (in soils, industrial effluents, groundwater) for a long period; easily bio accumulated and bio magnify within the food chains poses a significant threat to the consumer and pollution of water sources by potentially toxic metals became a worldwide problem [2]. The toxic effect of these metals could also be because of metabolic interference and mutagenesis. These metals interfere in the normal functioning of structural proteins, enzymes, and nucleic acids by binding them. Even a smaller amount of potentially toxic metals/metalloid arsenic, lead, cadmium, nickel, mercury, chromium, cobalt, and zinc beyond their permissible limit in body became harmful. These metals also enrich antibiotic resistant microbes even in the absence of antibiotics. This study discusses the health risks of potentially toxic metals contaminated water to the citizenry accumulated via intake of contaminated vegetables, fruits, fishes (freshwater or marine), drinking water, and beverages. The consequences of those metals on antibiotic resistant genes and bacteria have also been discussed.

2. Potentially toxic metals

Potentially toxic metals are essential in a small amount for various biochemical and physiological functions within the plants, animals, and humans. These metals participate in the redox reactions and are an important part of enzymes. A number of researchers [3–6] have reported that natural contaminates of natural water are potentially toxic metals and organometallic compounds. Based on their health importance, the potentially toxic elements are classified into four groups, (i) essential: Cu, Zn, Co, Cr, Mn, and Fe. These metals beyond their permissible limit become toxic, (ii) non-essential: Ba, Al, Li, (iii) less toxic: Sn, and (iv) highly toxic: Hg, Cd, Pb, As (metalloid).

2.1 Routes of uptake

Routes of uptake of those toxic metals by human and animals are:

i. Ingestion: it occurs via gastrointestinal route, that is, through the mouth by eating contaminated food, vegetables, fruits, seafood including fish, and by drinking contaminated water and beverages.

ii. Dermal: dermal uptake means absorption through skin/gills, the aquatic animals' bio accumulates these toxic metals via dermal contact.

iii. Inhalation: inhalation uptake occurs via inhalation of the polluted air as dust fumes and through exposure at work place. In the fish, these metals enter the body directly from water or sediments via the gills/skin or via its alimentary tract from the fish food/prey.

3. Sources of potentially toxic element contaminants within the water

Contamination of the environment by potentially toxic metals has increased after war II because of rapid industrialization and urbanization and increased rate of mobilization and transport [7]. The main sources of groundwater of contamination by heavy metals are:

3.1 Natural

Rock weathering, forest fires, volcanic eruptions, biogenic sources, and wind born soil particles are the natural sources of potentially toxic metals within the environment. Within the rocks, these metals are present as hydroxides, sulphides, oxides, silicates, phosphates, and chelated with organic compounds.

3.2 Anthropogenic activities

Industrial manufacturing of products to satisfy with the stress of the massive population like to cement production, iron industry, steam power plants, glass production, paint, and tanning industries is one among the causes of environmental pollution because of human activities. Agricultural activities (use of sewage sludge as manure), irrigation by sewage wastewater, mining, and metallurgical processes, garbage and waste mud incineration facilities, combustion of fuels, surface emission, and traffic and runoffs are other ways to release the pollutants within the different environmental compartments. The main route of the groundwater and aquatic contamination by potentially toxic metals are the leaching from toxic industrial waste dumps and municipal landfills and leaching of agricultural chemicals from soils into the upper aquifers [8].

As the concentration of potentially toxic metals within the environment is continuously increasing, and therefore, the soil retention capacity of those metals is decreasing and the resultant is the leaching of those metals within the groundwater [9]. Fertilizers and pesticides applied within the fields contain these potentially toxic metals (Cr, Cd, Cu, Zn, Ni, Mn, Pb, and As) as impurities [7]. Another source of groundwater contamination by potentially toxic metals is the urban runoffs which contain Pb, Cu, Zn, Fe, Cd, Cr, and Ni. The intrusion of seawater in aquifers also causes a rise in concentration levels of potentially toxic metals in the groundwater. Another anthropogenic source of the heavy metals in the environment is the burning of wastes at residential levels and dumpsites.

4. Potentially toxic metals within the ground, surface water, and sediments

The pollution of water resources by potentially toxic metals affects plants, animals, and human health adversely [10]. These metals even at a low concentration are toxic to aquatic organisms as these metals alter the histopathology of the tissues of the organisms [11, 12]. The one among the main sources of potentially toxic metals within the aquatic environment are the sediments which act as a sink and reservoir of those metals [13].

4.1 Potentially toxic metals within the drinking, ground, and surface water

A review of the literature showed that globally number of groundwater, drinking water, and surface water samples contains the potentially toxic metals beyond their permissible limit which affects adversely the human and ecological health. The arsenic concentration in the groundwater samples ranged from 0.0005 to 1.15 mg/L [14–16]. Author himself [17, 18] studied the concentration of potentially toxic metals in the groundwater samples for 20 years (1986–2005) and found that (i) concentration of those metals are increasing with time, (ii) concentration of those metals decreased with depth, and (iii) the concentration became beyond the permissible limit after the year 2000. The concentration of the toxic metals in the groundwater, drinking water, and surface water samples are recorded in **Table 1**.

4.2 Potentially toxic metals within the sediments

The accumulated amounts of the potentially toxic metals in the sediments are reported in **Table 1**.

5. Bioaccumulation of probably toxic metals in vegetables and fruits irrigated by contaminated ground and surface water

A long-term study made by the author himself [17, 18] found that the concentration of potentially toxic metals in the soils of agricultural fields of Aligarh irrigated by sewage effluent is continuously increasing, and therefore, the concentration of those metals in edible parts of the crops grown such soils were beyond toxic limits, and maximum accumulation was within the potato followed by maize [53]. Bansal [53] during their studies on the concentrations of Pb, Cd, Ni, Cr, Zn, and Cu in the vegetables palak, cabbage, brinjal, lady's finger, tomato, bitter gourd, radish, and cauliflower grown in the soils of periurban areas of Aligarh irrigated by sewage effluent water found that the concentration of the metals Cd, Pb, and Ni in all the studied vegetables were beyond their permissible limits for human consumption. The Target Hazard Quotient (THQ) values also denote that consumption of those vegetables will cause a potential risk for human health risk. Kabir and Bhuyan [54] found that the concentration of Cu in the hen's egg yolk (1.85–3.65 mg/kg) and albumin (0.5–1.15 mg/kg) were beyond permissible limits. The concentrations of these metals in the vegetables grown globally are given in **Table 1**.

6. Bioaccumulation of potentially toxic metals in freshwater fish, marine fish aqueous flora and fauna

Bioaccumulation of the potentially toxic heavy metals within the ecosystem of the Riverine has a negative impact on the ecological health of aquatic animals and causes decrease in their populations [55, 56]. Several researchers have reported fish deformities, decline of fish populations, and reduce in their growth rates if the concentration of potentially toxic metals increased beyond their tolerable limit [57, 58]. The concentrations of those metals in freshwater fish are reported in **Table 2**. The info in **Table 3** denotes the concentration of those metals in marine fish and other organisms.

Sample	Source	Concentration of metal (mg/L) or (mg/kg)								Reference
		Cd	Cr	Cu	Zn	Pb	Ni	As	Others	
Drinking water	Lagos state, Nigeria	0.0	0.009–0.021	0.027–0.060	0.11–0.41	0.098–0.14	0.72–1.02			[19]
Drinking water and surface water	Yobe State, Nigeria		0.0074–0.99	0.001–0.12	0.012–0.087	0.024	0.0			[20]
Surface water	Nile River and its canals	0.001–0.048				0.054–0.329				[21]
Drinking water	Egypt	0.002–0.049				0.09–0.41				
Drinking water	Nigeria	0.02–0.124;		0.009–0.057	0.08–20.1	0.04–0.57		0.091–0.485		[22]
Surface water	Pearl River, China	0.0005–0.0075	0.0035–0.011	0.003–0.005	0.0165–0.0607	0.0006–0.0011	0.0014–0.0045			[4]
Surface water	Dares salaam, Tanzania	0.32	0.59	0.03	1.14	0.46–0.55			0.99–1.26 (Fe)	[23]
Surface water	Ganga River, India	0.0–18.55	0.003–6.28	2.25–63.56	4.70	0.166–107.34	0.06–5.9	4.73		[5, 6, 24]
Ground water	Chembarambakkam lake (India)	0.00–1.32	0.00–0.19	0.018–0.088	0.008–2.45,	0.172–0.486	0.00–0.03			[25]
Surface water		0.00–1.5	0.00	0.01–0.03	0.01–0.70	0.16–0.22	0.00			
Surface water	Tamilnadu		0.229–1.484	0.001–0.128	0.001–0.65	0.031–0.781;	0.01–0.695			[26]
Surface water	Solan district (India)	0.00–0.00004			0.0021–0.0072	0.0 0–0.0041,		0.00–0.0014		[27]
Ground water		0.00001–0.00033			0.0006–0.0015	0.0001–0.0029		0.0–0.0009		
Surface water	Bodo Creek water	0.03–0.06				1.03–1.63				[28]
Surface water	Kenya	0.31–0.53		1.37–1.92		0.57–2.43				[29]

Sample	Source	Concentration of metal (mg/L) or (mg/kg)								Reference
		Cd	Cr	Cu	Zn	Pb	Ni	As	Others	
Ground water	Maru Town, Nigeria		0.0–0.99	0.0–0.33	0.012–0.087		0.00–0.0056			[30]
Groundwater	Albania	0.0–0.0006		0.0075–0.078		0.001–0.0058		0.008–0.009		[31]
Groundwater	Iran	0.006				0.09				[32]
Ground water	Singhbhum, India	0.01–0.08	0.04–0.28			0.08–0.42	0.03–0.14		0.07–4.45 (Fe)	[33]
Sediments	River Raohe, Chia	0.00–1.60	13.5–97.1	15.6–793.5	11.2–52.9	16.0–222.2	18.4–66.4	12.9–318.0		[13]
Sediments	Mashavera Basin Georgia	1.5–1.7	26.4–28	347.8–410.7	423.3–458.9	29.6–37.2	22.3–22.5		0.00–0.02 (Hg)	[34]
Sediments	Kabul	4.4–7.1	75.5–92.5	10.9–15.3	8.1–88.3	32.8–54.6	69.1–85.1			[35]
Sediments	River of Philippines		32.8–131.8	29.4–217.1	76.8–263.3		12.1–98.1		4.1–25.3 (Co)	[36]
Sediments	River Gomati	1.9–8.4		9.0–95.4		35.8–90.9		3.7–15.0		[37]
Sediments	River Ghaghara	0.21–0.28	61.3–84.7	2.8–11.7	13.3–17.6	10.7–14.3	15.3–25.6		11.4–18.4 (Co)	[38]
Sediments	River Ganga	1.7	69.9	29.8	67.8	26.7	26.7			[39]
Sediments	Bay of Bengal	0.03–0.06	0.61–0.79	0.38–0.66		0.01–1.42	0.01–0.23			[40]
Vegetables	Bangladesh	0.03–2.4	0.03–22.6	0.4–52.3	0.33–95.5	0.0.02–61.5	0.03–1.02	0.63–1.33	0.02–32 (Mn)	[41–43]
Vegetables	Supermarket of the Florida	0.002–0.040	0.012–0.223	0.13–2.47	1.31–3.95	0.0019–0.065	0.012–0.291	0.002–0.020	0.0005–0.033 (Co)	[44]
Vegetables		0.0006–0.028	0.009–0.126	0.22–2.65	1.12–3.88	0.0005–0.07	0.010–0.096	0.0012–0.016	0.0012–0.0065 (Co)	

Sample	Source	Concentration of metal (mg/L) or (mg/kg)								Reference
		Cd	Cr	Cu	Zn	Pb	Ni	As	Others	
Vegetables	Iran	0.030.55		0.85–4.1		0.5–1.5			0.69 (Co)	[45, 46]
Vegetables	Pakistan	0.045–0.39	2.72–6.62	22.2–65.2	19.5–41		1.8–5.0		18.7–137.3 (Mn)	[47]
Vegetables	Nigeria	0.11–0.43	5.1–9.9	4.7–75	38.1–335.2	2.6–9.2			19.3–33.3 (Mn)	[48]
Vegetables	Local vegetables, Iraq	1.5–6.0	1.02–1.13	7.3–37.2	25.3–43.8	0.5–1.48	6.3–7.9	4.73	2.83–3.09 (Co)	[49]
Vegetables	Imported vegetables, Iraq	1.6–5.8	1.03–1.15	17.3–33.5	17.3–33.5	0.32–1.55	7.1–10.3		3.08–3.10 (Co)	
Vegetables	China	0.004–0.51		0.015–1.31	1.4–24.2	0.004–1.16		0.014–0.66		[50]
Vegetables	Indonesia		0.0–152.8	4.3–150.1	5.1–90.7	11.1–347.5				[51]
Vegetables	Germany	0.01–0.79	0.03–4.69	3.2–23.2	11.7–122.8	0.1–31.3	0.03–1.93			[52]

Table 1.
The concentration of different potentially toxic metals (mg/L) in drinking, ground, and surface water and in sediments and vegetables (mg/kg).

Fish species	Source	Tissue	Concentration of metal (mg/kg)							Reference
			Cd	Cr	Cu	Zn	Pb	As	Hg	
Cyprinus carpio	Sardaryab, tributary of River Kabul	Gills		0.154	0.024	0.074	0.041			[59]
		Liver		0.188	0.089	0.07	0.142			
		Muscles		0.024	0.016	0.018	0.000			
Labeo rohita	Sardaryab, tributary of River Kabul	Gills		0.133	0.018	0.058	0.024			
		Liver		0.165	0.071	0.088	0.161			
		Muscles		0.019	0.01	0.02	0.000			
Cyprinus carpio	Indus River Mianwali, Pakistan	Gills		2.9–9.4	0.77–1.4	—	0.5–1.87			[60]
		Liver		3–5.4	2.5–3.4	—	0.45–1.1			
		Kidney		1.55–3.5	1.4–2.5	—	0.48–0.9			
		Muscles		1.03–2.63	1.1–1.67	—	0.46–1.9			
Wallago attu	Indus River Mianwali, Pakistan	Gills		4.5–9.5	3–5.9	—	0.45–1.92			
		Liver		12.5–20	11.5–21	—	0.9–1.0			
		Kidney		2.0–6.5	1.4–3.5	—	0.0–0.5			
		Muscles		6.5–15.2	2.9–5.5	—	0.83–2.0			
Labeo rohita	Kolleru Lake, India	Gills	0.38	0.19	0.09	0.19	0.3		0.05	[61]
		Liver	0.62	0.69	1.06	1.04	1.48		0.27	
		Kidney	0.25	0.72	0.23	0.94	0.55		0.07	
		Muscles	0.32	0.02	0.09	0.38	0.22		0.04	
Channa striatus	Kolleru Lake, India	Gills	0.32	0.59	0.03	1.14	1.30		0.12	
		Liver	0.48	0.33	0.99	1.01	1.35		0.20	
		Kidney	0.16	0.47	1.03	1.21	1.33		0.25	
		Muscles	0.45	0.85	0.53	0.46	1.30		0.14	

Fish species	Source	Tissue	Concentration of metal (mg/kg)							Reference
			Cd	Cr	Cu	Zn	Pb	As	Hg	
Oreochromis niloticus	Burullus Lake, Egypt	Muscles	0.45	0.85	0.39	4.70	0.46			[62]
Finfish	Lower Gangetic Delta, India	Whole Body	0–1.32		1.3–53.1	2.0–111.5	0–3.05			[63]
Shrimp	Lower Gangetic Delta, India	Whole Body	0–1.5		6.2–109.2	11.7–213.7	0–10			
Oyster	Lower Gangetic Delta, India	Whole Body	BDL		8.7–69.1	21.4–202.8	0–8			
Tilapia zillii	Niger River, Nigeria	Gill	0.094			8.92	ND		ND	[64]
		Muscle	0.049			5.42	ND		ND	
		Intestine	0.119			12.20	ND		ND	
Malapterurus electricus	Niger River, Nigeria	Gill	0.056			5.77	ND		ND	
		Muscle	0.032			3.74	ND		ND	
		Intestine	0.049			5.74	ND		ND	
Clarias gariepinus	Niger River, Nigeria	Gill	0.055			5.55	ND		ND	
		Muscle	0.04			3.38	ND		ND	
		Intestine	0.033			6.5	ND		ND	
Clarias batrachus	Local fish ponds of Ludhiana city and Sutlej River	Liver	3.74	3.69	3.48	67.78	11.12	3.13		[58]
		Muscle	0.24	2.10	3.79	29.42	4.48	0.68		
		Kidney	4.45	2.14	4.65	56.83	8.04	3.09		
Barbuss harpeyi	Tigris River in Baghdad	Gills	2.3–2.4	2.2–2.5	1.1–1.2	1.05–1.1	1.5–1.6			[65]
		Liver	1.3–2.9	2.5–2.7	0.5–0.8	0.9	2.05			
		Muscle	0.97–1.2	1.6–1.6	0.6–0.7	0.80	1.05			
Barbus xanthopterus	Bodo Creek, Niger Delta, Nigeria	Gills	2.2–2.5	2.1–2.5	1.2–1.3	1.1–1.2	1.3–1.6			
		Liver	2.7–2.8	2.2–2.6	0.7–0.8	0.7–0.9	1.8–2.1			
		Muscle	0.8	0.5–1.6	0.7–0.8	0.7–0.8	1.1			

Fish species	Source	Tissue	Concentration of metal (mg/kg)							Reference
			Cd	Cr	Cu	Zn	Pb	As	Hg	
Callinectes amnicola	Bodo Creek, Niger Delta, Nigeria	Leg	0.43–3.78				0.3–1.13			[27]
		Gill	0.38–2.02				0.01–0.42			
		Muscle	0.00–1.13				0.01–0.62			
		carapace	2.4–5.43				0.00–0.47			
Chrysichthys nigrodigitatus	Densu River, Ghana	Muscles			0.59	2.34		0.19	0.37	[11]
Alosa immaculata	Danube River	Whole Body	0.09		5.34		0.65			[66]
Cyprinus carpio	Danube River	Whole Body	0.084		5.10		0.58			
Cyprinus carpio	Danube River, Belgrade, Siberia	Whole Body	0.014		0.207		0.036			[67]
Silurus glanis	Danube River, Belgrade, Siberia	Whole Body	0.08		0.235		0.014			
Silurus glanis	Danube River	Whole Body	0.09		0.07		0.17	0.33		[68]
Sander lucioperca	Danube River	Whole Body	0.04		0.11		0.23	0.3		
Tilapia mossambica	Water bodies of Aurangabad, India	Gill		3.66–4.58	0.32–0.46					[69]
		Skin		1.80–2.74	0.19–0.26					
		Liver		1.56–2.16	0.29–0.36					
		Muscle		2.98–4.23	0.26–0.32					
Oreochromis niloticus	Lakes of Coimbatore, India	Muscle	1.26–1.59		8.49–9.69	18.38–25.94	5.91–9.69			[70]
		Gill	1.47–1.85		9.9–11.3	21.05–29.71	6.89–11.30			
		Liver	1.76–2.22		11.74–13.42	25.08–35.4	8.07–13.24			
Lutjanus griseus	Pearl Delta river China	Whole Body	0.03				0.03	0.39		[71]
Lutjanus stellatus	Pearl Delta river China	Whole Body	0.07				0.04	1.53		
Thunnus albacares	Egypt	Whole Body	0.06				0.32			[72]

Fish species	Source	Tissue	Concentration of metal (mg/kg)							Reference
			Cd	Cr	Cu	Zn	Pb	As	Hg	
Oncorhynchus mykiss	Hamadan Province, Iran	Whole Body	0.17–13.74				0.34–70.17			[73]
		Muscle	0.17–11.88				0.34–35.19			
		Liver	0.17–13.74				1.29–70.17			

Table 2.
The concentration of different potentially toxic metals in different parts of freshwater fish.

Fish species	Source	Tissue	Concentration of metal (mg/kg)							Reference
			Cd	Cr	Cu	Zn	Pb	As	Hg	
Mullet	Southeast Coast of Indian Ocean	Gills	0.013		0.092	0.087	0.043			[74]
		Gonad	0.001		0.192	0.284	0.302			
		Muscle	0.013		0.034	0.074	0.009			
		Skin	0.010		0.016	0.018	0.000			
		Whole Body	0.005		0.085	0.176	0.026			
Crab	Southeast Coast of Indian Ocean	Muscle	0.027		0.243	0.228	0.237			
		Gonad	0.060		0.330	0.244	0.150			
		Whole Body	0.004		0.061	0.259	0.013			
Shrimp	Southeast Coast of Indian Ocean	Skin	0.001		0.082	0.233	0.268			
		Whole Body	0.001		0.2	0.088	0.007			
Euthynnus affinis	Tok Bali Port, Malaysia	Whole Body	0.007		0.70	62.4	0.3			[57]
Pampus argenteus	Tok Bali Port, Malaysia	Whole Body	0.004		0.038	4.83	0.024			
Decapterus macrosoma	Tok Bali Port, Malaysia	Whole Body	0.003		0.064	5.29	0.001			
Leiognathus daura	Tok Bali Port, Malaysia	Whole Body	0.004		0.018	5.45	0.003			
Fenneropenaeus indicus	Tok Bali Port, Malaysia	Whole Body	0.04		0.34	14.4	0.008			
Lates calcarifer		Whole Body	0.007		0.49	6.5	0.20			[75]
Johnius belangerii	Red Sea, Jeddah Coast, Saudi Arabia	Whole Body			1.35	23.33	1.45			[76]
Chirocentrus dorab		Whole Body			1.45	22.91	1.0			
Arius maculatus		Whole Body			1.15	25.95	0.85			
Parastromateus niger		Whole Body			2.55	22.29	1.0			
Oyster	Gulf of Chabahar	Soft tissue	0.08–0.45	12.7–38.0	59.2–133.5	87–191	2.36–17.5			[77]

DOI: http://dx.doi.org/10.5772/intechopen.92141

Fish species	Source	Tissue	Concentration of metal (mg/kg)							Reference
			Cd	Cr	Cu	Zn	Pb	As	Hg	
Liocarcinus depurator	Samsun coasts of the Black Sea Turkey	Soft tissue	0.07		7.7	19	0.48			[78]
Rapana venosa		Soft tissue	0.085		4.3	9	0.12			
Mytilus galloprovincialis		Soft tissue	0.08		9.2	14	0.50			
Otolithes ruber	Persian Gulf, Iran	Soft tissue	0.21–0.47				1.98–2.98			[79]
Lutjanus johnii	Persian Gulf, Iran	Soft tissue	0.17–0.38				2.53–3.12			
Lagocephalus sceleratus	North-eastern Mediterranean part of Turkey	Muscle	0.045–0.139	0.20–0.36	0.276–0.518	51.4–86.63	1.46–2.56			[80]
		Skin	0.113–0.217	0.10–0.15	0.168–0.209	3.34–6.45	0.34–0.58			
Hirundichthys coromandelensis	Southeast coast of India	Soft tissue	0.02		0.26–0.28	3–3.28	0.20–0.24			[81]
Cypselurus spilopterus	Southeast coast of India	Soft tissue	0.02		0.26–0.33	2.15–3.30	017–0.19			
Sardina	Algerian coasts, Algeria	Soft tissue	0.55			2.13	0.62			[82]
Xiphias gladius	Algerian coast, Algeria	Soft tissue	0.57			3.90	0.56			
Brachydeuterus auritus	Fishing Habour Ghana,	Muscle			0.42	2.28		0.2	0.31	[11]
Pennahia anea	Coastal Waters, Malaysia	Muscle	0.03–0.21		0.94–4.38	17.7–26.3	0.14–0.41			[83]
		Liver	0.44–0.69		6.7–19.8	7–114.4	0.96–1.26			
		Gill	0.02–0.21		1.08–6.52	48.2–115.7	0.45–1.96			
Arius maculatus		Muscle	0.04–0.09		0.83–3.68	23–48.6	0.15–0.36			
		Liver	0.23–0.98		17.94–55	356–558	0.1–1.16			
		Gill	0.02–0.19		1.65–6.95	282–528	0.24–0.5			
Decapterus maraudsi	Terengganu Coastal Area, Malaysia	Soft tissue	0.2		0.64	7.97	0.17			[84]
Megalaspis cordyla	Terengganu Coastal Area, Malaysia	Soft tissue	0.31		1.16	10.42	0.02			
Bramidae	Terengganu Coastal Area, Malaysia	Soft tissue	1.53		0.98	15.14	0.09			

Fish species	Source	Tissue	Concentration of metal (mg/kg)							Reference
			Cd	Cr	Cu	Zn	Pb	As	Hg	
Selaroides leptolepis	Terengganu Coastal Area, Malaysia	Soft tissue	0.66		0.68	11.28	0.14			
Epinephelus lanceolatus	Terengganu Coastal Area, Malaysia	Soft tissue	0.64		0.83	12.51	0.11			
Rastrellige	Terengganu Coastal Area, Malaysia	Soft tissue	0.25		0.5	9.39	0.73			
Nibea soldado	Terengganu Coastal Area, Malaysia	Soft tissue	0.12		0.29	5.91	ND			
Pristipomoides filamentosus	Terengganu Coastal Area, Malaysia	Soft tissue	0.08		0.25	4.88	ND			
Priacanthus tayenus	Terengganu Coastal Area, Malaysia	Soft tissue	0.08		0.42	6.63	0.13			
Siganus canaliculatus	Terengganu Coastal Area, Malaysia	Soft tissue	0.10		0.68	11.60	0.15			
Thunnus obesus	Western and Central pacific ocean	Soft tissue							0.929	
Trichiurus lepturus	Coastal Waters of Ondo State, Nigeria	Muscle	0.0	0.0	0.0	0.34	0.09			[85]
		Head	0.21	0.32	0.0	0.38	0.20			
		Eye	0.37	0.35	0.0	0.38	0.20			
		Gill	0.48	0.49	0.87	0.51	0.15			
		Bone	0.32	0.35	0.59	0.10	0.12			
Pentanmius guigarius		Muscle	0.0	0.0	0.58	0.35	0.1			
		Head	0.26	0.37	0.0	0.36	0.34			
		Eye	0.49	0.62	0.0	0.65	0.14			
		Gill	1.14	1.28	1.88	1.29	0.40			
		Bone	0.32	0.38	0.59	0.39	0.11			
Pseudotolithus senegalensis		Muscle	0.0	0.0	0.46	0.36	0.10			
		Head	0.27	0.26	0.38	0.38	0.71			
		Eye	0.29	0.32	0.39	0.39	0.04			

Fish species	Source	Tissue	Concentration of metal (mg/kg)							Reference
			Cd	Cr	Cu	Zn	Pb	As	Hg	
		Gill	0.81	0.86	0.94	0.94	0.27			
		Bone	0.31	0.38	0.39	0.39	0.12			
Pseudotolithus typus		Muscle	0.31	0.36	0.0	0.36	0.07			
		Head	0.28	0.23	0.0	0.38	0.16			
		Eye	0.30	0.37	0.0	0.39	0.01			
		Gill	0.32	0.37	0.62	0.42	0.12			
		Bone	0.32	0.37	0.59	0.38	0.11			
Cyprinus carpio L,	Ala gul wetland (Iran)	Muscle	0.0–0.140		1.23–39.4	1.15–47.7	0–21.86			[86]
Cyprinus carpio L,	Alma gul wetland (Iran)		0.0–0.02		1.23–4.4	19.15–117.4	2.1–8.7			

Table 3.
The concentration of different potentially toxic metals in different tissues of marine organisms.

7. Potentially toxic metals-resistance

The potentially toxic metals (Cd, Cu, Pb, Zn, Cr (III), Cr (VI), and Hg) aren't only toxic to human health but also enrich antibiotic resistant microbes particularly bacteria. Co-selection of an antibiotic and metal resistance in bacteria is extremely important because it promotes antibiotic resistance in bacteria even in the absence of antibiotics. Co-selection occurs by two mechanisms:

i. Co-resistance: when antibiotics and these metals co-exist within the same environment, these metals influence some antibiotic resistant bacteria to survive in more polluted environment. Co-resistance occurs when two or more different resistant genes are present on the same genetic elements (plasmid, transposon, Integron) or are present within the same bacterial strain which provides resistant to different compounds. The rise of antibiotic resistant genes is directly correlated with the concentration of those metals [87].

ii. Cross-resistance: cross resistance occurs when antibiotics and potentially toxic metals target the same microbes leading to generic detoxification of genes by reducing intracellular concentration of antibiotics and metals, and enhanced efflux occurs during cross-resistance [87].

Besides these two mechanisms, co-selection is additionally promoted by co-regulatory mechanism which occurs when different resistant genes is controlled by one regulator gene [88]. The impact of the potentially toxic metals on the antibiotic resistant bacterial strain is a given in **Table 4**.

8. Toxicity of potentially toxic metals

World Health Organization has reported that globally in the year 2015 approximately 8.8 million deaths were due to cancer, presence of potentially toxic metals beyond permissible limits within the environment is one among the main factors of the death because the endocrine system is disrupted by these metals. When the food or drinking water containing potentially toxic metals beyond their maximum tolerance concentration is ingested, the metabolism of living cells in the body is negatively affected [122]. The immune and hematopoietic systems in human and animals also are adversely affected on exposure to the mixtures of those metals [122]. Li et al. [123] reported that the main cause for human bone diseases is the presence of the potentially toxic metals beyond their permissible limit within the aquatic environment. Potentially toxic metals Pb, Hg, Cd, As, and Cr in living cells causes cytotoxicity [124] and oxidative stress [124], leading to the damages of antioxidants, enzyme inhibition, apoptosis (programmed cell death), loss of DNA repair mechanism, protein dysfunction, and damage to lipid peroxidase and of the membrane.

8.1 Cadmium

Cadmium in human causes Itai-Itai disease, liver/kidney lesions, hepato-colic effects [125], carcinoma, prostatic adenocarcinoma, osteoporosis, hypertension, disorder, and kidney lesions including enlargement, nuclear, and mitochondrial damages, and histological changes; decreased antioxidant power of kidney also

Toxic metal	Mechanism of action	Mechanism of resistance	Antibiotic categories / generic names	Pathogen(s)
Cu	Produces hyperoxide radicals by interaction with cell membrane. Enzymatic activities are inhibited and cellular functions are disrupted.	Resistant genes are located on plasmids and transposons and transfers in between bacterial species.	Tetracycline	*Klebsiella* spp. [89, 90]; *Fecal Enterococci* [91]; *E. coli* [92]; *E. faecium* [93]
			Carbapenem	*Pseudomonas aeruginosa* [94]
			Vancomycin, Amphenicol	*Enterococcus faecium* [93, 95]
			Chloramphenicol	*Bacillus* spp. isolated from ship [96]
			Erythromycin	soil bacteria of Scotland [90]; *Enterococcus faecium* [95]
			Fluoroquinolone	*E. coli* [92]; *E. faecium* [93]
			Quinolone; Sulphonamide	*E. coli* [92]
			Cephalosporin	*Fecal Enterococci* [91]
			Penicillin; Cephalosporin; Nitrofuran	*Enterobacter* spp.; *P. aeruginosa* [97]
			Macrolide	*E. faecium* [98]
Hg	Hg inactivates the enzymatic activities, interferes in the protein synthesis and DNA function, and disrupts cell membrane. Destroys the biological membranes as the mercuric ions are lipid soluble so easily passed through biological membranes.	Hg resistant genes are located on plasmids and transposons. The resistance mechanism involves the reduction of Hg^{2+} ions to Hg in the cytoplasm of the bacteria by the enzyme mercuric reductase which is encoded with the merA gene.	Sulphonamide, Chloramphenicol, Ampicillin, Streptomycetin, Augmentin	*Salmonella enterica* [99]; Fecal Gram-negative bacteria [100]
			Fluoroquinolone, Quinolone	*E. coli*, *Citrobacter* spp., Klebsiella spp. [101]
			Penicillin	*Salmonella* spp. [102]; *Serratia* spp. [103]
			Tetracycline	*E. coli*; *Citrobacter* spp.; *Klebsiella* spp. [104]; *E. faecium* [105]
			Teicoplanin	*Salmonella* spp. [102]
			Sulphonamide; Cephalosporin; Macrolide	*E. coli*; *Citrobacter* spp.; *Enterobacter* spp.; *Klebsiella* spp.; *Proteus* spp. [106]
			Cephalosporin	*E. coli* [107]; *Citrobacter* spp.; *Enterobacter* spp.; *Klebsiella* spp.; *Proteus* spp. [106]

Toxic metal	Mechanism of action	Mechanism of resistance	Antibiotic categories / generic names	Pathogen(s)
			Aminoglycoside	*E. coli*; *Citrobacter* spp.; *Enterobacter* spp.; *Klebsiella* spp.; *Salmonella* spp.; *P. aeruginosa* [108]
			Vancomycin	*E. faecium* [100]
Zn	Due to affinity of Zn to thiol group, the Zn metal is toxic to bacteria, retards glycolysis, transmembrane proton translocation and acid tolerance in the bacterial cell. Also decreases the biomass causing growth inhibition.	Resistance to Zn is found in Gram negative and gram positive bacteria and resistance is mainly via *czr*C gene	Norfloxacin, Augmentin, Gentamicin, Ampicillin	Bacteria isolated from the soil of Kenya [109]
			Carbapenem	*Pseudomonas aeruginosa* [94]
			Penicillin, Teicoplanin	*Salmonella* spp. [102]
			Fluoroquinolone, quinolone	*E. coli*; *Citrobacter* spp. [101]
			Methicillin	*Staphylococcus aureus* [110]
Cr	Due to strong oxidizing potential the metal Cr damages the cells of the microbes,inhibits the oxygen uptake, growth and elongation of lag phase.	Cr in microbes affects basal energy metabolism, protein oxidative stress protection, DNA repair, detoxification of enzymes, efflux pumps, homeoostasis	Tetracycline, Carbapenem	Soil bacteria of Scotland [90]
			Penicillin	*Enterobacter* spp. [97]
			Cephalosporin, Tetracycline	*P. aeruginosa* [97]
			Nitrofuran, Teicoplanin	*Salmonella* spp. [102]
			Quinolone, Vancomycin	*E. coli* [111]
			Sulfonamide	*Klebsiella* spp. [112]
Cd	Cd in bacteria denatures the protein, interacts with calcium metabolism, damages the cell membrane, hinders cell division and transcription, and also affects the nucleic acid.	Resistance to Cd in Gram negative bacteria affects Czc and Ncc genes and encoding dsbA gene needed for disulphite formation while in Gram positive bacteria resistance to Cd is with the CdA pump	Augmentin, Ampicillin	Bacteria isolated from the soil of Kenya [109]
			Ampicillin	Bacteria isolated from ship [96]
			Fluoroquinolone, Quinolone	*E. coli*; *Citrobacter* spp.; *Klebsiella* spp. [101]
			Penicillin, Tetracycline	*P. aeruginosa* [113]
			Amphenicol, Cephalosporin Methicillin, Sulfonamide, Aminoglycoside	*E. coli*; *Citrobacter* spp.; *Klebsiella* spp. [112]
			Macrolide	*E. faecium* [98]

Toxic metal	Mechanism of action	Mechanism of resistance	Antibiotic categories / generic names	Pathogen(s)
Pb	Lead induces mutagenicity, inhibits enzyme activities and transcription. Pb in the bacteria destroys the nucleic acid.	Resistance mechanism is due to adsorption of lead by extracellular polysaccharides, cell exclusion and ion efflux to the cell exterior.	Aminoglycoside	*Citrobacter* spp. [104]
			Macrolide, Quinolone	*E. coli* [111]
			Penicillin	*Enterobacter* spp. [107]
			Teicoplanin	*E. faecium* [105]
			Quinolone	*Klebsiella* spp. [106]
			Sulphonamide	*Proteus* spp. [106]
			Vancomycin	*Enterobacter* spp.; *Klebsiella* spp. [106]
			Amphenicol	*Salmonella* Spp. [114]
			Fluoroquinolone	*P. aeruginosa* [115]
			Tetracycline	*Shigella* spp. [116]
Ni	Ni replaces the essential metals from metalloprotein. The activity of the enzymes is retarded as Ni binds the catalytic site of the enzyme. Ni causes oxidative stress which results in the enhanced DNA damage, protein impairment, and lipid peroxidation.	The resistance mechanism is due to energy-dependent Ni efflux pump induced by cnr which is promoted by a chemo-osmotic proton-antiporter system.	Quinolone	*E. coli* [111]
			Tetracycline	Soil bacteria of Scotland [90]
			Penicillin	*Salmonella* spp. [102]
			Amphenicol	*E. faecium* [105]
			Sulfonamide	*Citrobacter* spp. [112]
As	Disrupts enzymatic functions in the cell and interferes in the phosphate uptake and utilization.	Activation of efflux pumps due to cross resistance between arsenic and antibiotics is the main mechanism	Penicillin	*E. coli* [107]
			Sulfonamide	*Salmonella* spp. [117]
			Tetracycline	*E. coli* [118]
			Amphenicol	*Salmonella* spp. [119]
Co	Produces non B_{12} cobalt protein.	The gene Czc, affects the inner and outer membranes and removes the cobalt from the cytoplasm	Aminoglycoside	*Citrobacter* spp. [106]
			Macrolide	*Enterobacter* spp. [120]
			Penicillin	*Salmonella* spp. [102]
			Quinolone	*E. coli* [111]
			Sulfamethoxazole	*P. aeruginosa* [121]
			Vancomycin	*Enterobacter* spp.; *Klebsiella* spp. [106]

Table 4.
Impact of potentially toxic metals on some bacterial strain resistant to antibiotics.

disrupts mineral balance within the body, causing dysfunctions of sexual glands and skeltel diseases. A psychomotor function of the brain is bogged down in the presence of Cd. The toxicity of cadmium to cell is because Cd can displace vitamin C and E from their metabolically active sites, decrease in absorption of calcium by intestine and enhanced dissolution of bone calcium causing disorder in the normal bone metabolism processes. Cd an endocrine disrupter causes neuro-developmental toxicity. Toxicity of Cd in fishes includes immune suppression and immune dysfunction.

8.2 Lead

Out of about four million tons of lead used per annum globally about three million tons is discharged within the environment. In the physical body, 90–95% of the intruding lead is accumulated within the bones which combine with bone minerals and organic matter causes rise in the blood lead level. Accumulation of lead within the bones affects the acid-base equilibrium causing calcium deficiency. Pb within the body lowers the active vitamin D_3 level and parathyroid level within the plasma affecting somatic cell function viz., decrease in the secretion of γ-carboxyglutamic acid containing protein. Clinical studies have shown that if the extent of Pb in the drinking water is 50 μg/L, the blood lead level within the human is going to be about 30 μg/L; if the extent increased further, the lead level within the breast fed babies are enhanced causing hindrance within the bone development. If the blood lead level in children exceeds 75 μg/L, it causes coma, convulsions, and eventually death. Pb also affects central systema nervosum, renal, cardiovascular, neurological, and musculoskeletal systems. Pb influences the heme synthesizing enzymes by replacing Zn within the heme synthesis. Lead disrupts biosynthesis of hemoglobin, metabolism of Fe, Zn, and Cu, and of vitamin D within the body, and also causes cognitive impairment. Pb in physical body also acts as nephrotoxicants. Lead in fish's body also affects immune system [122]. Long-term exposure to the low concentration of a mix of Cd, As, and Pb in human and other animal cause hepatotoxic (damage to the liver) effects [123].

8.3 Chromium

The annual output of Cr globally is approximately 7.5 million tons. The secretion of Collagen-Type I which helps in the bone fracture healing is suppressed in the presence of chromium ion. Chromium in human causes nose ulcers, asthma, DNA damage, hemolysis, damage to liver, kidney, and carcinoma.

8.4 Arsenic

Smith et al. [126] after their research studies reported that if the person get 50 μg/L of arsenic (daily) then 13 out of 1000 individuals will suffer with lung, liver, kidney or bladder cancer. Skin lesions are by the uptake of 0.0012 mg/kg/day of arsenic. Bhattacharya et al. [125] found that low concentration of arsenic for long period damages liver in human and other animals. Enlargement of kidney, nuclear, and mitochondrial damages, histological changes, and decreased antioxidant power of kidney is additionally caused by arsenic in human. Arsenic also causes neurotoxic effects in human with the assembly of the reactive oxygen species which incorporates death of neuronal cells, cognitive dysfunction, and Alzheimer's disease. Cognitive impairment, deafness, hypertension, anemia dementia, hematemesis, and bladder cancer also is caused by As. The prolonged exposure to arsenic also affects central systema nervosum.

8.5 Mercury

Mercury is the third top hazardous substance. Aquatic organisms convert inorganic mercury to methyl mercury which inactivates Na+/K+ ATPase. Hg with the production of reactive oxygen causes neurotoxic effects in human including death of neuronal cells, cognitive dysfunction, and Alzheimer's disease. As Hg is an endocrine disrupter, during pregnancy exposure to metal causes long-term damages to new born as mercury disrupts the influences the maternal-fetal balance. Minamata disease, renal toxicity, skin, nose irritation, damage to central systema nervosum, hearing speech, and visual disorders are another health risks to human.

8.6 Copper

Copper an integral part of several enzymes in small amount (0.9 mg daily uptake) is an essential metal for animals and plants. Deficiency of copper in human causes anemia, a low number of leucocytes, defects in animal tissue, and osteoporosis in infants. The copper within the body beyond its permissible limit causes hematemesis, jaundice, melena, damage to central nervous system, liver, and kidney problems. Wilson's disease a genetic disease is additionally caused by copper.

8.7 Nickel

Nickel, a natural occurring metal, exists in a number of mineral forms and is an ingredient of chocolate, steel, and other metal products, pigments, valves and of batteries. Excess uptake of nickel by human causes asthma, pneumonia, allergies, heart disorder, skin rashes, and miscarriage. Chances of development of carcinoma, nose cancer, larynx cancer, and prostatic adenocarcinoma also are enhanced.

8.8 Cobalt

Cobalt is an essential metal for the life as it is the integral part of vitamin B_{12} (cobalamin). Human when exposed to the higher concentration of cobalt causes decreased pulmonary function, asthma, interstitial lung disease, wheezing, and dyspnoea and reduces pulmonary function. Respiratory tract hyperplasia, pulmonary fibrosis, increase in number of red blood cells, emphysema, paralysis of the systema nervosum, seizures, growth retardation, and thyroid deficiency are diseases occurs in human at a really high concentration of the metal.

8.9 Zinc

As zinc plays a crucial role in number of metallo enzymes viz., dehydrogenase, alkaline phosphatase, carbonic anhydrase, leucine amino peptidase, superoxide dismutase, and deoxyribosenucleic acid (DNA) and ribosenucleic acid (RNA) polymerase is an essential metal in humans and animals. Over exposures to zinc in human causes dry or pharyngitis, chest tightness, headache, increased indices of pulmonary inflammation, nausea, decrease in the activity of copper metallo enzyme, decreased HDL-cholesterol level, immuno toxicity, and gastrointestinal effects.

9. Conclusions

- Contamination of ground and surface water by potentially toxic metals is a worldwide problem.
- The major route of the groundwater and aquatic contamination by potentially toxic metals are the leaching from toxic industrial waste dumps, municipal landfills, and leaching of agricultural chemicals from soils into the upper aquifers.
- Potentially toxic metals contaminated vegetables and fruits; fishes, seafood, and drinking water are the most sources of the ingestion of those metals by the citizenry.
- A number of biological and biochemical processes are disrupted in the physical body by accumulation of those metals. These metals also cause developmental abnormalities in the children.
- These potentially toxic metals promote the spread of antibiotic resistant genes which causes the ineffectiveness of broad- spectrum antibiotics.

Declaration

No original data is utilized in this review; all information is accessed from published work.

Author details

Om Prakash Bansal
Chemistry Department, D.S. College, Aligarh, India

*Address all correspondence to: drop1955@gmail.com

IntechOpen

© 2020 The Author(s). Licensee IntechOpen. This chapter is distributed under the terms of the Creative Commons Attribution License (http://creativecommons.org/licenses/by/3.0), which permits unrestricted use, distribution, and reproduction in any medium, provided the original work is properly cited.

References

[1] Li L, Yang X. The essential element manganese, oxidative stress, and metabolic diseases: Links and interactions. Oxidative Medicine and Cellular Longevity. 2018;**2018**:7580707. DOI: 10.1155/2018/.580707

[2] Zwolak A, Sarzyńska M, Szpyrka E, Stawarczyk K. Sources of soil pollution by heavy metals and their accumulation in vegetables: A review. Water, Air, and Soil Pollution. 2019;**230**:164. DOI: 10.1007/s11270-019-4221-y

[3] Ali H, Khan E, Ilahi I. Environmental chemistry and ecotoxicology of hazardous heavy metals: Environmental persistence, toxicity, and bioaccumulation. Journal of Chemistry. 2019;**2019**:6730305. DOI: 10.1155/2019/6730305

[4] Jiao Z, Li H, Song M, Wang L. Ecological risk assessment of heavy metals in water and sediment of the Pearl River estuary, China. Materials Science and Engineering. 2018;**394**: 052055. DOI: 10.1088/1757-899X/394/5/052055

[5] Nizami G, Rehman S. Assessment of heavy metals and their effects on quality of water of rivers of Uttar Pradesh, India: A review. Environmental Toxicology and Chemistry. 2018;**2**:65-71

[6] Paul D. Research on heavy metal pollution of river ganga: A review. Annals of Agrarian Science. 2017;**15**: 278-286

[7] Toth G, Hermann T, Da Silva MR, Montanerella L. Heavy metals in agricultural soils of the European Union with implications for food safety. Environment International. 2016;**88**: 299-309

[8] Sharma B, Sarkar A, Singh P, Singh RP. Agricultural utilization of biosolids: A review on potential effects on soil and plant grown. Waste Management. 2017;**64**:117-132. DOI: 10.1016/j.wasman.2017.03.002

[9] Galitskaya IV, Rama Mohan K, Keshav Krishna A, Batral GI, Eremina ON, Putilina VS, et al. Assessment of soil and groundwater contamination by heavy metals and metalloids in Russian and Indian megacities. Procedia Earth and Planetary Science. 2017;**17**:674-677

[10] Rezania S, Taib SM, Md Din MF, Dahalan FA, Kamyab H. Comprehensive review on phytotechnology: Heavy metals removal by diverse aquatic plants species from wastewater. Journal of Hazardous Materials. 2016;**318**:587-599

[11] Gbogbo F, Arthur-Yartel A, Bondzie JA, Dorleku WP, Dadzie S, Kwansa-Bentum B, et al. Risk of heavy metal ingestion from the consumption of two commercially valuable species of fish from the fresh and coastal waters of Ghana. PLoS One. 2018;**13**(3):e0194682. DOI: 10.1371/journal.pone.0194682

[12] Ahmed MK, Parvin E, Islam MM, Akter MS, Khan S, Al-Mamun MH. Lead- and cadmium-induced histopathological changes in gill, kidney and liver tissue of freshwater climbing perch *Anabas testudineus* (Bloch, 1792). Chemistry and Ecology. 2014;**30**: 532-540

[13] Wei J, Duan M, Li Y, et al. Concentration and pollution assessment of heavy metals within surface sediments of the Raohe Basin, China. The Scientific Reporters. 2019;**9**:13100. DOI: 10.1038/s 415 98-019-49724-7

[14] Kulkarni HV, Mladenov N, Datta S, Chatterjee D. Influence of monsoonal recharge on arsenic and dissolved organic matter in the Holocene and Pleistocene aquifers of the Bengal Basin.

Science of the Total Environment. 2018; **637–638**:588-599. DOI: 10.1016/j.scitonev.2018.05.009

[15] Fatima S, Hussain I, Rasool A, Xiao T, Farooqi A. Comparison of two alluvial aquifers shows the probable role of river sediments on the release of arsenic in the groundwater of district Vehari, Punjab, Pakistan. Environmental Earth Sciences. 2018;**77**: 382. DOI: 10.1007/s12665-018-7542-z

[16] Jiang Z, Li P, Tu J, Wei D, Zhang R, Wang Y, et al. Arsenic in geothermal systems of Tengchong, China: Potential contamination on freshwater resources. International Biodeterioration & Biodegradation. 2018;**128**:28-35. DOI: 10.1016/j.ibiod.2016.05.013

[17] Bansal OP. Groundwater quality of Aligarh district of Uttar Pradesh, India, a 11 year study. Pollution Research. 2008;**27**:721-724

[18] Bansal OP. Heavy metals in soil, plants as influenced by irrigation with sewage effluents: A 20 year study. Journal of Indian Association for Environmental Management. 2008;**35**: 143-148

[19] Chika OC, Prince EA. Comparative assessment of trace and heavy metals in available drinking water from different sources in the Centre of Lagos and off town (Ikorodu LGA) of Lagos state, Nigeria. Advanced Journal of Chemistry, Section A. 2020;**3**(1):94-104

[20] Kwaya MY, Hamidu H, Kachalla M, Abdullahi IM. Preliminary ground and surface water resources trace elements concentration, toxicity and statistical evaluation in part of Yobe State, North Eastern Nigeria. Geosciences. 2017;**7**:117-128. DOI: 10.5923/j.geo.20170704.02

[21] Salman SA, Zeid SAM, Seleem EMM, Abdel-Hafiz MA. Soil characterization and heavy metal pollution assessment in Orabi farms, El Obour, Egypt. Bulletin of the National Research Centre. 2019;**43**:42. DOI: 10.1186/s42269-019-0082-1

[22] Aloke C, Uzuegbu IE, Ogbu PN, Ugwuja EL, Orinya OF, Obasi IO. Comparative assessment of heavy metals in drinking water sources from Enyigba Community in Abakaliki Local Government Area, Ebonyi state, Nigeria. African Journal of Environmental Science and Technology. 2019;**13**:149-154

[23] Kacholi DS, Sahu M. Levels and health risk assessment of heavy metals in soil, water, and vegetables of Dar es Salaam, Tanzania. Journal of Chemistry. 2018;**2018**:1402674. DOI: 10.1155/2018/1402674

[24] Chakraborti D, Singh S, Rahman M, Dutta R, Mukherjee S, Pati S, et al. Groundwater arsenic contamination in the Ganga River basin: A future health danger. International Journal of Environmental Research and Public Health. 2018;**15**:180. DOI: 10.3390/ijerph15020180

[25] Ramachandran A, Krishnamurthy RR. Jayaprakash M, Balasubramanian M: Concentration of heavy metal in surface water and groundwater Adyar River basin, Chennai, Tamilnadu, India. IOSR Journal of Applied Geology and Geophysics. 2018; **6**:29-35

[26] Sridhar SGD, Sakthivel AM, Sangunathan U, Jenefer S, Mohamed Rafik M, Kanagaraj G. Heavy metal concentration in groundwater from Besant Nagar to Sathankuppam, South Chennai, Tamil Nadu, India. Applied Water Science. 2017;**7**:4651-4662

[27] Rana A, Bhardwaj SK, Thakur M, Verma S. Assessment of heavy metals in surface and ground water sources under different land uses in mid-hills of Himachal Pradesh. International Journal of Bio-resource and Stress Management.

2016;7(3):461-465. DOI: 10.5958/0976-4038.2016.00074.9

[28] Godwin AOM, Chinenye NG. Bioaccumulation of selected heavy metals in water, sediment and blue crab (*Callinectes amnicola*) from Bodo Creek, Niger Delta, Nigeria. Journal of Fisheries Science. 2016;**10**(3):77-83

[29] Wasike PW, Nawiri MP, Wanyonyi AA. Levels of heavy metals (Pb, Mn, Cu and Cd) in water from river Kuywa and the adjacent wells. Environment and Ecology Research. 2019;7:135-138. DOI: 10.13189/eer.2019.070303

[30] Kwaya MY, Hamidu H, Mohammed I, Abdulmumini N, Adamu IH, Grema M, et al. Heavy metals pollution indices and multivariate statistical evaluation of groundwater quality of Maru town and environs. Journal of Materials and Environmental Science. 2019;**10**:32-44

[31] Deda A, Alushllari M, Mico S. Measurement of heavy metals in ground water. AIP Conference Proceedings. 2019;**2109**:100001-100004. DOI: 10.1063/1.5110136

[32] Vatandoosta M, Naghipoura D, Omidia S, Ashrafia SD. Survey and mapping of heavy metals in groundwater resources around the region of the Anzali international wetland; a dataset. Data in Brief. 2018;**18**:463-469

[33] Singh UK, Ramanathan AL, Subramanian V. Groundwater chemistry and human health risk assessment in the mining region of east Singhbhum Jharkhand, India. Chemosphere. 2018;**204**:501-513. DOI: 10.1016/j.chemosphere.2018.04.060

[34] Withanachchi SS, Ghambashidze G, Kunchulia I, Urushadze T, Ploeger A. Water quality in surface water: A preliminary assessment of heavy metal contamination of the Mashavera River, Georgia. International Journal of Environmental Research and Public Health. 2018;**15**(4):621. DOI: 10.3390/ijerph15040621

[35] Khan MI, Khisroon M, Khan A, Gulfam N, Siraj M, Zaidi F, et al. Bioaccumulation of heavy metals in water, sediments, and tissues and their histopathological effects on Anodonta cygnea (Linea, 1876) in Kabul River, Khyber Pakhtunkhwa, Pakistan. BioMed Research International. 2018;**2018**:1910274. DOI: 10.1155/2018/1910274

[36] Decena SCP, Arguilles MS, Robel LL. Assessing heavy metal contamination in surface sediments in an Urban River in the Philippines. Polish Journal of Environmental Studies. 2018;**27**(5):1983-1995. DOI: 10.15244/pjoes/75204

[37] Neha Kumar D, Shukla P, Kumar S, Bauddh K, Tiwari J, Dwivedi N, et al. Metal distribution in the sediments, water and naturally occurring macrophytes in the river Gomti, Lucknow, Uttar Pradesh, India. Current Science. 2017;**113**:1578-1585

[38] Singh H, Pandey R, Singh SK, Shukla DN. Assessment of heavy metal contamination in the sediment of the river Ghaghara, a major tributary of the river ganga in northern India. Applied Water Science. 2017;7:4133-4149

[39] Pandey J, Singh R. Heavy metals in sediments of Ganga River: Up- and downstream urban influences. Applied Water Science. 2017;7:1669-1678

[40] Khan MZH, Hasan MR, Khan M, Aktar S, Fatema K. Distribution of heavy metals in surface sediments of the Bay of Bengal coast. Journal of Toxicology. 2017;**2017**:9235764. DOI: 10.1155/2017/9235764

[41] Uddin MN, Hasan MK, Dhar PK. Contamination status of heavy metals in vegetables and soil in Satkhira,

Bangladesh. Journal of Materials and Environmental Science. 2019;**10**:543-552

[42] Ratul AK, Hassan M, Uddin MK, Sultana MS, Akbor MA, Ahsan MA. Potential health risk of heavy metals accumulation in vegetables irrigated with polluted river water. International Food Research Journal. 2018;**25**(1):329-338

[43] Sultana MS, Rana S, Yamazaki S, Aono T, Yoshida S. Sofian Kanan (reviewing editor): Health risk assessment for carcinogenic and non-carcinogenic heavy metal exposures from vegetables and fruits of Bangladesh. Cogent Environmental Science. 2017;**3**:1. DOI: 10.1080/23311843.2017.1291107

[44] Hadayat N, De Oliveria L, Silva ED, Han L, Hussain M, Liu X, et al. Assessment of trace metals in five most-consumed vegetables in the US: Conventional vs. organic. Environmental Pollution. 2018;**243**:292-300

[45] Naghipour D, Chenari MA, Taheri N, Naghipour F, Mehrabian F, Attarchi MA, et al. The concentration data of heavy metals in vegetables of Guilan province, Iran. Data in Brief. 2018;**21**:1704-1708

[46] Zafarzadeh A, Rahimzadeh H, Mahvi AH. Health risk assessment of heavy metals in vegetables in an endemic esophageal cancer region in Iran. Health Scope. 2018;**7**(3):e12340. DOI: 10.5812/jhealthscope.12340

[47] Latif A, Bilal M, Asghar W, Azeem M, Ahmad IM, Abbas A, et al. Heavy metal accumulation in vegetables and assessment of their potential health risk. International Journal of Environmental Analytical Chemistry. 2018;**5**(1):234-245. DOI: 10.4172/2380-2391.1000234

[48] Hong AH, Umaru AB. Heavy metals concentration levels in vegetables irrigated from Lake Geriyo area of Adamawa state, Nigeria. International Journal of Engineering and Science Invention. 2018;**7**:39-42

[49] Hassoon HA. Heavy metals contamination assessment for some imported and local vegetables. Iraqi Journal of Agricultural Sciences. 2018; **49**(5):794-802

[50] Zhou H, Yang WT, Zhou X, Liu L, Gu JF, Wang WL, et al. Accumulation of heavy metals in vegetable species planted in contaminated soils and the health risk assessment. International Journal of Environmental Research and Public Health. 2016;**13**:289-296. DOI: 10.3390/ijerph13030289

[51] Siaka IM, Utama IMS, Manuaba IBP, Adnyana M. Heavy metals contents in the edible parts of some vegetables grown in Candi Kuning, Bali and their predicted pollution in the cultivated soil. Journal of Environment and Earth Science. 2014;**4**:78-83

[52] Säumel I, Kotsyuk I, Hölscher M, Lenkereit C, Weber F, Kowarik I. How healthy is urban horticulture in high traffic areas? Trace metal concentrations in vegetable crops from plantings within inner city neighborhoods in Berlin, Germany. Environmental Pollution. 2012;**165**:124-132. DOI: 10.1016/j.envpol.2012.02.019

[53] Bansal OP. Heavy metals in sewage effluent water irrigated vegetables and their potential health risks to consumers of Aligarh, India. Chemical Science Review and Letters. 2014;**3**:589-596

[54] Kabir A, Bhuyan MS. Heavy metals in egg contents of hens (Gallus gallus domesticus) and ducks (Anas platyrhynchos) from Chittagong region. Bangladesh Journal Pollution Effective Control. 2019;**7**:232-237

[55] Malik DS, Maurya PK. Heavy metal concentration in water, sediment, and tissues of fish species (Heteropneustis

fossilis and Puntius ticto) from Kali River, India. Toxicological & Environmental Chemistry. 2014;**96**: 1195-1206

[56] Luo J, Ye Y, Gao Z, Wang W. Essential and nonessential elements in the red-crowned crane *Grus japonensis* of Zhalong wetland, North-Eastern China. Toxicological & Environmental Chemistry. 2014;**96**:1096-1105

[57] Salam MA, Paul SC, Noor SNBM, Siddiqua SA, Aka TD, Wahab R, et al. Contamination profile of heavy metals in marine fish and shellfish. Global Journal of Environmental Science and Management. 2019;**5**:225-236

[58] Kaur S, Khera KS, Kondal JK. Effect of water contaminated with heavy metals on histopathology of freshwater catfish, *Clarias batrachus*. International Journal of Chemical Studies. 2018;**6**(4): 3103-3108

[59] Yousafzai AM, Ullah F, Bari F, Raziq S, Riaz M, Khan K, et al. Bioaccumulation of some heavy metals: Analysis and comparison of *Cyprinus carpio* and *Labeo rohita* from Sardaryab, Khyber Pakhtunkhwa. BioMed Research International. 2017;**2017**:5801432. DOI: 10.1155/2017/5801432

[60] Mahoob S, Kausar S, Jabeen F, Sultana S, Sultana T, Al-Ghanim KA, et al. Effect of heavy metals on liver, kidney, gills and muscles of *Cyprinus carpio* and *Wallago attu* inhabited in the Indus. Brazilian Archives of Biology and Technology. 2016;**59**:1-10. DOI: 10.1590/1678-4324-20161502

[61] Harsimran Kaur B. Accumulation of heavy metals in fishes of freshwater [Thesis]. Department of Zoology, University of Delhi; 2016. p. 44

[62] El-Batrawy OA, El-Gammal MI, Mohamadein LI, Darwish DH, El-Moselhy M. Impact assessment of some heavy metals on tilapia fish, *Oreochromis niloticus*, in Burullus Lake, Egypt. The Journal of Basic and Applied Zoology. 2018;**79**:13. DOI: 10.1186/s41936-018-0028-4

[63] Ray Chaudhuri T, Dutta P, Zaman S, Mitra A. Status of edible fishes of lower gangetic delta in terms of heavy metals. International Journal of Environmental Sciences & Natural Resources. 2017;**5**(3):555661. DOI: 10.19080/IJESNR.2017.05.555661

[64] Ibemenuga KN, Ezike F, Nwosu MC, Anyaegbunam LC, Okoye EI, Eyo JE. Bioaccumulation of some heavy metals in some organs of three selected fish of commercial importance from Niger River, Onitsha shelf, Anambra state, Nigeria. Journal of Fisheries Science. 2019;**13**:001-012

[65] Mensoor M, Said A. Determination of heavy metals in freshwater fishes of the Tigris River in Baghdad. Fishes. 2018;**3**:23. DOI: 10.3390/fishes3020023

[66] Ionita C, Mititelu M, Morosan E. Analysis of heavy metals and organic pollutants from some Danube River fishes. Farmácia. 2014;**62**(2):299-305

[67] Milanov DR, Krstic M, Markovic R, Jovanovic AD, Baltic MB, Ivanovic SJ, et al. Analysis of heavy metals concentration in tissues of three different fish species included in human diet from Danube River, in the Belgrad region, Serbia. Acta Veterinaria Belgrade. 2016;**66**:89-102

[68] Miloskovic A, Dojcinovic B, Kovacevic S, Radojkovic N, Radenkovic M, Milosevic D, et al. Spatial monitoring of heavy metals in the inland waters of Serbia: A multispecies approach based on commercial fish. Environmental Science and Pollution Research. 2016;**23**(10):9918-9933

[69] Khillare K, Khillare YK, Wagh U. Bioaccumulation of heavy metals in freshwater fishes from Aurangabad

district Maharashtra. World Journal of Pharmacy and Pharmaceutical Sciences. 2015;**4**:511-520

[70] Mercy M, Dhanalakshmi B. Toxicological evaluation of heavy metals in tissues of freshwater fish *Oreochromis niloticus* collected from lakes of Coimbatore district, Tamilnadu, India. International Research Journal of Pharmacy. 2017;**8**(1):41-45. DOI: 10.7897/2230-8407.08018

[71] Leung HM, Leung AO, Wang HS, Ma KK, Liang Y, Ho KC, et al. Assessment of heavy metals/metalloid (As, Pb, Cd, Ni, Zn, Cr, Cu, Mn) concentrations in edible fish species tissue in the Pearl River Delta (PRD), China. Marine Pollution Bulletin. 2014; **78**(1–2):235-245. DOI: 10.1016/j. marpolbul.2013.10.028

[72] El-Moselhy KM, Othman AI, El-Azem A, El-Metwally MEA. Bioaccumulation of heavy metals in some tissues of fish in the Red Sea, Egypt. Egyptian Journal of Basic and Applied Sciences. 2014;**1**:97-105

[73] Reyahi-Khoram M, Setayesh-Shiri F, Cheraghi M. Study of the heavy metals (Cd and Pb) content in the tissues of rainbow trouts from Hamedan Coldwater fish farms. Iranian Journal of Fisheries Sciences. 2016;**15**(2):858-869

[74] Sulieman HMA, Suliman EAM. Appraisal of heavy metal levels in some marine organisms gathered from the Vellar and Uppanar estuaries southeast coast of Indian Ocean. Journal of Taibah University for Science. 2019;**13**: 338-343

[75] Nasyitah SN, Ahmad ZA, Khairul NM, Ley JL, Kyoung-Woong K. Bioaccumulation of heavy metals in Maricultured fish, *Lates calcarifer* (Barramudi), *Lutjanus campechanus* (red snapper) and *Lutjanus griseus* (Grey snapper). Chemosphere. 2018;**197**: 318-324. DOI: 10.1016/j. chemosphere. 2017.12.187

[76] Younis AM, Amin HF, Alkaladi A, Mosleh YYI. Bioaccumulation of heavy metals in fish, squids and crustaceans from the Red Sea, Jeddah coast, Saudi Arabia. Open Journal of Marine Science. 2015;**5**:369-378. DOI: 10.4236/ ojms.2015.54030

[77] Bazzi AO. Heavy metal in sea water, sediment and marine organism in the gulf of Chabahar, Oman Sea. Journal of Oceanography and Marine Science. 2014;**5**:20-29

[78] Bat L, Arici E, Sezgin M, Sahin F. Heavy metals in edible tissues of benthic organisms from Samsun coasts, south Black Sea Turkey and their potential risk to human health. Journal of Food and Health Science. 2016;**2**:57-66. DOI: 10.3153/JFHS16006

[79] Sadeghi E, Pirsaheb M, Mohammadi M, Salti AP, Sharafi H, Mirzaei N, et al. Evaluation of cadmium and lead levels in fillet marine fish (*Otolithes ruber and Lutjanus johni*) from Persian gulf. Annals of Tropical Medicine & Public Health. 2017;**10**: 1015-1018

[80] Eken M, Aydin F, Turan F, Uyan A. Bioaccumulation of some heavy metals on silver-cheeked toadfish (*Lagocephalus sceleratus*) from Antalya Bay, Turkey. Natural and Engineering Sciences. 2017;**2**(3):12-21

[81] Jayaprabha N, Balakrishnan S, Purusothaman S, Indira K, Srinivasan M, Anantharaman P. Bioaccumulation of heavy metals in flying fishes along southeast coast of India. International Food Research Journal. 2014;**21**(4):1381-1386

[82] Mehouel F, Bouayad L, Hammoudi AH, Ayadi Q, Regad F. Evaluation of the heavy metals (mercury, lead, and cadmium)

contamination of sardine (*Sardina pilchardus*) and swordfish (*Xiphias gladius*) fished in three Algerian coasts. Veterinary World. 2019;**12**(1):7-11. DOI: 10.14202/vetworld.2019.7-11

[83] Bashir FA, Alhemmali EM. Analysis of some heavy metal in marine fish in muscle, liver and gill tissue in two marine fish spices from Kapar coastal waters, Malaysia. In: The Second Symposium on Theories and Applications of Basic and Biosciences. Misrata, Libya; 2015

[84] Rosli MNR, Samat SB, Yasir MS, Yusof MFM. Analysis of heavy metal accumulation in fish at Terengganu coastal area, Malaysia. Sains Malaysiana. 2018;**47**(6):1277-1283. DOI: 10.17576/jsm-2018-4706-24

[85] Olusola JO, Festus AA. Assessment of heavy metals in some marine fish species relevant to their concentration in water and sediment from coastal waters of Ondo state, Nigeria. Journal of Marine Science: Research & Development. 2015;**5**:163. DOI: 10.4172/2155-9910.1000163

[86] Bandpei AM, Bay A, Zafarzadeh A, Hassanzadeh V. Bioaccumulation of heavy metals muscle of common carp fish (Cyprinus carpio L, 1758) from Ala gul and Alma gul wetlands of Golestan and consumption risk assessment. International Journal of Medical Research & Health Science. 2016;**5**:267-273

[87] Tugui C, Szekeres E, Baricz A. Sources and mechanisms of combined heavy-metal and antibiotic resistance traits in bacteria. Studia Universitatis Babeş-Bolyai Biologia. 2017;**LXII**: 101-114

[88] Pal C, Asiani K, Arya S, Rensing C, Stek DJ, DGJ L, et al. Metal resistance and its association with antibiotic resistance. Advances in Microbial Physiology. 2017;**70**:261-301. DOI: 10.1016/bs.ampbs.2017.02.001

[89] Knapp CW, Callan AC, Aitken B, Shearn R, Koenders A, Hinwood A. Relationship between antibiotic resistance genes and metals in residential soil samples from Western Australia. Environmental Science and Pollution Research International. 2017; **24**(3):2484-2494. DOI: 10.1007/s11356-016-7997-y

[90] Knapp CW, McCluskey SM, Singh BK, Campbell CD, Hudson G, Graham DW. Antibiotic resistance gene abundances correlate with metal and geochemical conditions in archived scottish soils. PLoS One. 2011;**6**:e27300. DOI: 10.1371/journal.pone.0027300

[91] Amachawadi RG, Scott HM, Alvarado CA, et al. Occurrence of the transferable copper resistance gene *tcrB* among fecal enterococci of U.S. feedlot cattle fed copper-supplemented diets. Applied and Environmental Microbiology. 2013;**79**:4369-4375

[92] Becerra-Castro C, Machado RA, Vaz-Moreira I, Manaia CM. Assessment of copper and zinc salts as selectors of antibiotic resistance in gram-negative bacteria. The Science of the Total Environment. 2015;**530-531**:367-372. DOI: 10.1016/j.scitotenv.2015.05.102

[93] Silverira E, Freitas AR, Antunes P, Barros M, Campos J, Coque TM, et al. Co-transfer of resistance to high concentrations of copper and first-line antibiotics among *Enterococcus* from different origins (humans, animals, the environment and foods) and clonal lineages. Journal of Antimicrobial Chemotherapy. 2014;**69**:899-906. DOI: 10.1093/jac/dkt479

[94] Li H, Luo YF, Williams BJ, Blackwell TS, Xie CM. Structure and function of OprD protein in *Pseudomonas aeruginosa*: From antibiotic resistance to novel therapies. International Journal of Medical Microbiology. 2012;**302**:63-68. DOI: 10.1016/j.ijmm.2011.10.001

[95] Wales AD, Davies RH. Co-selection of resistance to antibiotics, biocides and heavy metals, and its relevance to foodborne pathogens. Antibiotics. 2015; **4**(4):567-604

[96] Kacar A, Kocyigit A. Characterization of heavy metal and antibiotic resistant bacteria isolated from Aliaga ship dismantling zone, eastern Aegean Sea, Turkey. International Journal of Environmental Research. 2013;**7**(4):895-902

[97] Heck K, De Marco ÉG, Duarte MW, Salamoni SP, Van Der Sand S. Pattern of multiresistant to antimicrobials and heavy metal tolerance in bacteria isolated from sewage sludge samples from a composting process at a recycling plant in southern Brazil. Environmental Monitoring and Assessment. 2015;**187**: 328. DOI: 10.1007/s10661-015-4575-6

[98] Vignaroli C, Pasquaroli S, Citterio B, Di Cesare A, Mangiaterra G, Fattorini D, et al. Antibiotic and heavy metal resistance in enterococci from coastal marine sediment. Environmental Pollution. 2018;**237**:406-413

[99] Baker-Austin C, Wright MS, Stepanauskas R, McArthur JV. Co-selection of antibiotic and metal resistance. Trends in Microbiology. 2006;**14**(4):176-182

[100] Ji X, Shen Q, Liu F, Ma J, Xu G, Wang Y, et al. Antibiotic resistance gene abundances associated with antibiotics and heavy metals in animal manures and agricultural soils adjacent to feedlots in Shanghai, China. Journal of Hazardous Materials. 2012;**235–236**: 178-185

[101] Anssour L, Messai Y, Estepa V, Torres C, Bakour R. Characteristics of ciprofloxacin-resistant Enterobacteriaceae isolates recovered from wastewater of an Algerian hospital. Journal of Infection in Developing Countries. 2016;**10**(07):728-734

[102] Ali NM, Mazhar SA, Mazhar B, Imtiaz A, Andleeb S. Antibacterial activity of different plant extracts and antibiotics on pathogenic bacterial isolates from wheat field water. Pakistan Journal of Pharmaceutical Sciences. 2017;**30**(4):1321-1325

[103] Mirzaei N, Rastegari H, Kargar M. Antibiotic resistance pattern among gram negative mercury resistant bacteria isolated from contaminated environments. Jundishapur Journal of Microbiology. 2013;**6**(10):634-639

[104] Habi S, Daba H. Plasmid incidence, antibiotic and metal resistance among enterobacteriaceae isolated from Algerian streams. Pakistan Journal of Biological Sciences. 2009;**12**(22): 1474-1482. DOI: 10.3923/pjbs.2009. 1474.1482

[105] De Niederhäusern S, Bondi M, Anacarso I, Iseppi R, Sabia C, Bitonte F, et al. Antibiotics and heavy metals resistance and other biological characters in *Enterococci* isolated from surface water of Monte Cotugno Lake (Italy). Journal of Environmental Science and Health, Part A. 2013;**48**(8): 939-946

[106] Djouadi LN, Selama O, Abderrahmani A, Bouanane-Darenfed A, Abdellaziz L, Amziane M, et al. Multiresistant opportunistic pathogenic bacteria isolated from polluted rivers and first detection of nontuberculous mycobacteria in the Algerian aquatic environment. Journal of Water and Health. 2017;**15**(4):566-579

[107] Verma T, Ramteke PW, Garg SK. Occurrence of chromium resistant thermotolerant coliforms in tannery effluent. Indian Journal of Experimental Biology. 2004;**42**(11):1112-1116

[108] Martins VV, Zanetti MOB, Pitondo-Silva A, Stehling EG. Aquatic environments polluted with antibiotics and heavy metals: A human health

hazard. Environmental Science and Pollution Research International. 2014; **21**(9):5873-5878

[109] Budambula NML, Kinyua DM. Antibiotic resistance of metal tolerant bacteria isolated from soil in Juja, Kenya. In: Conference Paper: JKUAT Scientific, Technological and Industrialization Conference November 2013. Nairobi; 2013

[110] Cavaco LM, Hasman H, Stegger M, Andersen PA, Skov R, Fluit AC, et al. Cloning and occurrence of czrC, a gene conferring cadmium and zinc resistance in methicillin-resistant Staphylococcus aureus CC398 isolates. Antimicrobial Agents and Chemotherapy. 2010;**54**(9): 3605-3608. DOI: 10.1128/AAC.00058-1

[111] Abskharon RN, Hassan SH, Gad El-Rab SM, Shoreit AA. Heavy metal resistant of *E. coli* isolated from wastewater sites in Assiut City, Egypt. Bulletin of Environmental Contamination and Toxicology. 2008; **81**(3):309-315

[112] Sepahy AA, Sharifian S, Zolfaghari MR, Dermany MK, Rashedi H. Study on heavy metal resistant fecal coliforms isolated from industrial, urban wastewater in Arak, Iran. International Journal of Environmental Research. 2015; **9**(4):1217-1224

[113] Deredjian A, Colinon C, Brothier E, Favre-Bonte S, Cournoyer B, Nazaret S. Antibiotic and metal resistance among hospital and outdoor strains *of Pseudomonas aeruginosa*. Research in Microbiology. 2011;**162**(7):689-700. DOI: 10.1016/j.resmic.2011.06.007

[114] Mourão J, Marçal S, Ramos P, Campos J, Machado J, Peixe L, et al. Tolerance to multiple metal stressors in emerging non-typhoidal MDR *Salmonella* serotypes: A relevant role for copper in anaerobic conditions. The Journal of Antimicrobial Chemotherapy. 2016;**71**(8):2147-2157

[115] Soltan MES. Isolation and characterization of antibiotic and heavy metal-resistant *Pseudomonas aeruginosa* from different polluted waters in Sohag district, Egypt. Journal of Microbiology and Biotechnology. 2001;**11**(1):50-55

[116] Manegabe BJ, Marie-Médiatrice NK, Barr Dewar J, Christian SB. Antibiotic resistance and tolerance to heavy metals demonstrated by environmental pathogenic bacteria isolated from the Kahwa River, Bukavu town, Democratic Republic of the Congo. International Journal of Environmental Studies. 2017; **74**(2):290-302

[117] Sandegren L, Linkevicius M, Lytsy B, Melhus A, Andersson DI. Transfer of an *Escherichia coli* ST131 multiresistance cassette has created a *Klebsiella pneumoniae*-specific plasmid associated with a major nosocomial outbreak. Journal of Antimicrobial Chemotherapy. 2012;**67**:74-83. DOI: 10.1093/jac/dkr40.5

[118] Gilmour MW, Thomson NR, Sanders M, Parkhill J, Taylor DE. The complete nucleotide sequence of the resistance plasmid R478: Defining the backbone components of incompatibility group H conjugative plasmids through comparative genomics. Plasmid. 2004;**52**:182-202

[119] Seginkova Z, Kralikova K. Monitoring the contemporary resistance of *Escherichia coli* and *Salmonella* Sp. strains isolated from aquatic environment to antibiotics and ions of heavy-metals. Ekologia Bratislava. 1993; **12**(1):111-118

[120] Hu Q, Dou MN, Qi HY, Xie XM, Zhuang GQ, Yang M. Detection, isolation, and identification of cadmium-resistant bacteria based on PCR-DGGE. Journal of Environmental Sciences. 2007;**19**(9):1114-1119

[121] Oyetibo GO, Ilori MO, Adebusoye SA, Obayori OS,

Amund OO. Bacteria with dual resistance to elevated concentrations of heavy metals and antibiotics in Nigerian contaminated systems. Environmental Monitoring and Assessment. 2010;**168**(1–4):305-314

[122] Ojedokun AT, Bello OS. Sequestering heavy metals from wastewater using cow dung. Water Resources and Industry. 2016;**13**:7-13

[123] Li JJ, Li-Na P, Shan W, Meng-Da Z. Advances in the effect of heavy metals in aquatic environment on the health risks for bone. Earth and Environmental Science. 2018;**186**:012057. DOI: 10.1088/1755-1315/186/3/012057

[124] Hernández-García A, Romero D, Gómez-Ramírez P, María-Mojica P, Martínez-López E, García-Fernández AJ. In vitro evaluation of cell death induced by cadmium, lead and their binary mixtures on erythrocytes of common buzzard (*Buteo buteo*). Toxicology In Vitro. 2014;**28**:300-306. DOI: 10.1016/j.tiv.2013.11.005

[125] Bhattacharya PT, Misra SR, Mohsina Hussain M. Nutritional aspects of essential trace elements in oral health and disease: An extensive review. Scientifica. 2016;**2016**:5464373. DOI: 10.1155/2016/5464373

[126] Smith AH, Lingas EO, Rahman M. Contamination of drinking-water by arsenic in Bangladesh: A public health emergency. Bulletin of the World Health Organization. 2000;**78**(9):1093-1103

Chapter 6

Toxicologic Characteristics of Nanodisperse Manganese Oxide: Physical-Chemical Properties, Biological Accumulation, and Morphological-Functional Properties at Various Exposure Types

Nina Vladimirovna Zaitseva
and Marina Alexandrovna Zemlyanova

Abstract

Nanosized manganese oxide has excellent prospects. Some data imply that its particles can be toxic when introduced in various ways, and it requires further examination of this nanomaterial. The authors conducted research of nanodisperse MnO_2 water suspension at intragastric, inhalation, and skin-resorptive introduction into small rodents and obtained profound characteristics of its toxic effects, determined target organs and revealed dose-dependent effects. The substance was characterized with acute toxicity, and its bioaccumulation under long-term exposure caused morphofunctional disorders in brain, lipid peroxidation activation, and lower antioxidant system activity. The authors detected vessel hyperemia, subarachnoid hemorrhages, brain edema with perivascular and pericellular spaces dilatation, nerve fiber demyelinization, and focal dystrophic changes in vessels endothelium. After a long-term introduction in doses from 0.25 to 2.5 mg/kg, oxidizing-antioxidant imbalance occurred, neurotransmitters and electrolytes balance was violated, and there was also brush border epithelium insufficiency. Nanodisperse MnO_2 water suspension in doses equal to 2.5 and 0.25 mg/kg at intragastric introduction into Wistar rats did not have embryotoxic or teratogenic effects. It did not have any mutagenic effects in doses equal to 10.3 and 5.15 mg/kg or gonadotoxic effects either when introduced into Wistar male rats in doses equal to 10.3–5.15 mg/kg via gastric tube.

Keywords: nanodisperse magnesium oxide, toxicity, acute exposure, chronic exposure, long-term effects, inhalation and oral route

1. Introduction

Nowadays, one can see rapid growth in worldwide development and commercialization of nanoindustries and nanotechnological products in overall production chain; such products and technologies are considered to belong to a market segment of new technologies (the sixth technological structure) [1]. As per US Congressional Research Service experts assessment, world market of finished products and goods containing nanocomponents and nanomaterials now amounts to more than 1 trillion US dollars; it comprises more than 800 consumer goods produced with the use of nanotechnologies; by 2020, more than 15% of overall goods output in the world will be produced with the use of nanodevelopments, and the volume of this market in various sectors will be equal to more than 3 trillion US dollars. Aggregate volume of investment into scientific research and start-ups related to nanotechnologies received from various sources worldwide is estimated to amount to almost 20 billion US dollars. Annual nanoindustries market growth is expected to reach 20–30% [2]. In experts' opinion, nanoindustries and nanotechnologies (together with other technologies) are already facilitating transfer to new technological structure based on renewable energy sources, intellectual power engineering technologies, construction of completely new energy-efficient buildings, hydrogen technologies application, electrical and hybrid vehicle creation, 3D printer design and implementation, etc.

Nowadays, nanoclusters evolve quite intensely all over the world (more than 1700 cluster organizations in 260 European regions) and in Russia (more than 330 participating organizations). World market segments of nanomaterials develop as their commercial use in such key spheres as aerospace, health care, biotechnologies, power engineering, electronics and IT, processing industries, and consumer goods sector, grows rapidly [1, 3]. All this becomes apparent in the attitudes the European Union (EU) has toward the matter, declaring that nanotechnology is one of the Key Emerging Technologies 2020 Strategy. Its enormous potential for innovation has fostered large investments in developing new consumer products and industrial applications. The outlooks for a rapid growth in the sector have raised not only hopes and high expectations, but also societal concerns about the adequacy of nanotechnology regulation. Indeed, despite their clear benefits, engineered nanomaterials pose environmental and health risks [4].

All these processes prove the necessity to systematically examine potential dangers and threats for human activity, which are related to large-scale spread of nanotechnologies and nanobiotechnologies. In spite of all their undeniable innovative properties, nanomaterials including those containing metal nanoparticles may cause certain health risk at all stages of production and product consumption due to their specific physical-chemical properties. They may also be dangerous for human environment objects and lead to grave social and economic consequences.

The challenges that researchers encountered provoked the need to develop reliable methods for characterization of nanoparticles released from various product matrices into complex biological, environmental and food media, and for the assessment of their human and environmental exposure, hazard, and risk [4]. Special attention is paid to detecting correlation between physical properties (i.e., size, shape, surface structure, and aggregation degree) of nanomaterials and toxic response induction in biological structures. This research direction has been actively developed in Federal Scientific Center for Medical and Preventive Health Risk Management Technologies (Perm) for many years. Physical properties of a number of widely spread metal-oxide nanoparticles as well as peculiarities of their biological and toxic effects exerted at various exposure types have not been studied sufficiently; so the research goal is to systemize the knowledge on the subject and to make it more precise.

2. Utilization prospects for nanosized particles of manganese oxide and sources of their introduction into environment

Nanosized particles of manganese oxide (MnO_2) represent a prospective nanomaterial, which can be used for creating high-technology components applicable in nanoelectronics, nano-optics, and nanochemistry [5]. Nowadays, nanodisperse MnO_2 is used as an active component in portable power sources, solar batteries, electrical appliances, accelerators, and sorbents [6, 7]. A possibility to use threadlike nanosized particles of MnO_2 for sensor electrodes creation is of particular interest for researchers [7]. Planned production of matrices based on nanosized MnO_2 for nanomagnetic materials and sorbents, nanoaccelerators, and semiconductor thermistors, can reach up to 1000 tons per year and is considered to be "mass production" [8]. Here, direct exposure of workers involved in the production process, as well as population living in areas influenced by such production, becomes quite possible. A possibility that the substance is introduced into the atmosphere in the form of aerosol is determined by technological processes as nanoparticles of MnO_2 are emitted in their course. Such processes include vacuum-ultrasound laser ablation applied in producing matrices of nanomagnetic materials and sorbents [9]. Laser ablation in suspension of nanodisperse MnO_2 includes local impulse-continuous heating of the substance, sublimation, crystallization, and hydrodynamic processes, which cause formation of nanodisperse MnO_2 aerosol.

Formation of nanodisperse MnO_2 aerosol occurs in production of sensory electrodes, biosensors, [6], cathode accelerators, and semiconductor thermistors [7], when electrochemical deposition is applied; this process means covering graphite rods with stable hydrosol of disperse MnO_2 nanoparticles in electroplating baths. Sewage formed in the processes contains MnO_2, and they can get into surface wells. Today, aerosol of nanodisperse MnO_2 can be found in civil engineering and chemical production facilities. Working area air at a production facility manufacturing potash fertilizers was examined; the research results proved that MnO_2 particles were present in the air; thus, there were about 4435–7330 million/m^3 particles sized 45–95 nm at a carrier driver workplace in a milling workshop (MnO_2 content in working area air was equal to 0.3 mg/m^3). Nanoparticles sized 5–25 nm in concentrations equal to 4588–11,423 million/m^3 were registered at a machine operator workplace in a granulating workshop. Manganese particles were identified among those nanoparticles via mass-spectrometry technique with inductive-bound plasma; Agilent 7500cx mass-spectrometer with octopole reaction collision cell was applied (Agilent Technologies Inc., USA) [10]. There are some data implying that MnO_2 particles can be toxic when introduced in various ways, and it requires further examination of this nanomaterial.

Detailed research on nanosized particles toxicity involves a wide range of tasks according to the recommendations set forth by Good laboratory practice (GLP): toxicology evaluation, single dose, repeated dose, toxicokinetics, genotoxicity, reproductive and developmental toxicology, and local toxicity. According to these recommendations, the authors have assessed toxicity of nanosized MnO_2. All the animals before the experiment underwent 14-day quarantine and were placed in standard cages made of polypropylene, two animals in each. Cages were in a ventilated room. Air temperature in the room was constant and equal to 23.0 ± 2.0°C, and air humidity was 60.0 ± 5.0%. The animals received semisynthetic nutrition with food and biological value, which completely satisfied all physiological needs. They also had free access to food and water. All procedures and examinations on animals were performed in full conformity with guide for the care and use of laboratory animals (ILAR, DELS) [11] and requirements set forth by Ethics Committee of Federal Scientific Center for Medical and Preventive Health Risk Management Technologies.

3. Results and discussion

3.1 Physical and chemical properties of nanodisperse magnesium oxide

The following substances were tested during the experiment: water suspension of nanodisperse magnesium oxide (III, IV) (manganese (III, IV) oxide, CAS Registry Number 1313-13-09). IUPAC name: manganese oxide and manganese (III, IV) oxide. Synonyms: manganese dioxide, manganese binoxide, and manganese peroxide [12].

According to the results of studying the particle size and shape with independent methods, it is found that the MnO_2 sample tested was a nanomaterial. This is evidenced by the study results of the water suspension test sample (MnO_2 concentration is 36.0 ± 2.3 mg/cm^3) with a residual CTAB in the suspension below the detection threshold (0.00001 mg/cm^3). The particle size distribution (cross-sectional dimension determined with dynamic laser light scattering) is represented in the bar chart as follows: 13 nm (1.2% of the total number of particles), 15–29 nm (94.4% of the total number of particles), and 33–100 nm (4.1% of the total number of particles). The maximum peak value of the particle size made 19 ± 4 nm (41.2% of the total number of particles) (**Table 1**).

Scanning electron microscopy revealed that the particles being visualized exceeded 20 nm in size. The difference with the previous method may be due to a failed focus of the scanning microscope on the nanoparticles smaller than 20 nm, despite sensitivity of 3–10 nm, as stated in its data sheet. As seen in particles are of filamentary shape (97.8% of the total number of particles). The determined sizes and the shape of particles are confirmed by atomic force microscopy (**Figures 1** and **2**).

The textural characteristics of resulting material studied showed that the adsorption-desorption isotherm of nitrogen corresponds to the type IV (isotherm with a distinct capillary condensation), and the shape of the hysteresis loop belongs to H3 type with the distinct area of mesopores filling within the range of relative pressures (p/p_0) 0.7–1. In other words, mesopores filling at higher relative pressures verifies the presence of large diameter mesopores (**Figure 3**).

The maximum pore size distribution occurs in the range of ~10 nm. The specific surface area (S_{BET}) of the nanosized particles, calculated by Brunauer et al. [13], amounted to 150.2 ± 2.6 m^2/g. The total pore volume was equal to 0.676 cm^3/g (the total pores volume (V_{tot}) was calculated from the amount of nitrogen adsorbed at a relative pressure $p/p0 \approx 0.99$. Pore size distribution was determined by the desorption isotherms by Barrett et al. [14]).

The water suspension of nanodisperse magnesium oxide had the following physicochemical characteristics: chemical formula: MnO_2, smiles: O=Mn=O, molar mass: 6.9368 g/mol, chemical composition of the nanosized phase: metal, presence of solvent: matrix-bidistilled water, particle charge: neutral at pH = 7.4, resistance to aggregation: particles are prone to aggregation, hydrophobicity: hydrophilic substance, Bp at 76 mm Hg: 3127°C, Bm: 1080°C; vapor tension (mm Hg) and volatility (mg/m^3 20°C): undetermined, specific weight: 4.8 g/cm^3, water solubility: insoluble, oil/water ratio: undetermined, and aggregation state: in water at 20 and 35°C—dark brown solid substance, in air at 20 and 35°C—dark brown powder, of high strength and hardness.

Size of particles in a suspension, micron	Proportion of particles, %
0.0131	1.2
0.0150	9.6
0.0171	16.4
0.0196	20.0
0.0225	21.2
0.0257	13.9
0.0295	13.2
0.0338	0.44
0.0387	0.38
0.0443	0.64
0.0507	0.90
0.0581	0.73
0.0666	0.42
0.0762	0.39
0.0873	0.15

Table 1.
Distribution of MnO_2 nanoparticles in a water suspension versus particle size using dynamic light scattering analyzer Horiba LB-550 (Horiba, Japan) [14].

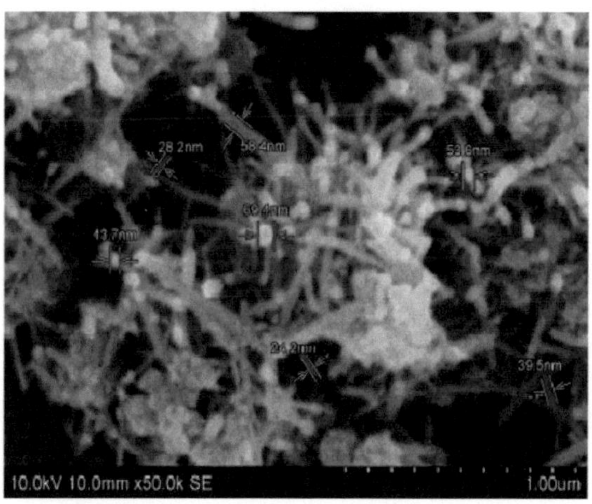

Figure 1.
Scanning electron microscopy image of MnO_2 nanoparticles, electron microscopy with a high-resolution scanning microscope (3–10 nm, max magnification of 300,000X) S-3400 N (Hitachi, Japan) with energy dispersive X-ray attachment for microanalysis (Bruker, Germany) [15].

3.2 Acute toxicity study of nanodisperse manganese oxide at various types of introduction into a body

3.2.1 Acute toxicity study of MnO_2 nanoparticles under inhalation exposure

Over the last decade, a lot of researchers have dedicated their work to practical application of a priority nanomaterial, namely, nanodisperse MnO_2 [16]. They are particularly interested in examining possibilities to use threadlike nanosized MnO_2 particles for sensory electrodes creation [6, 7] or cathode accelerator creation [7] at

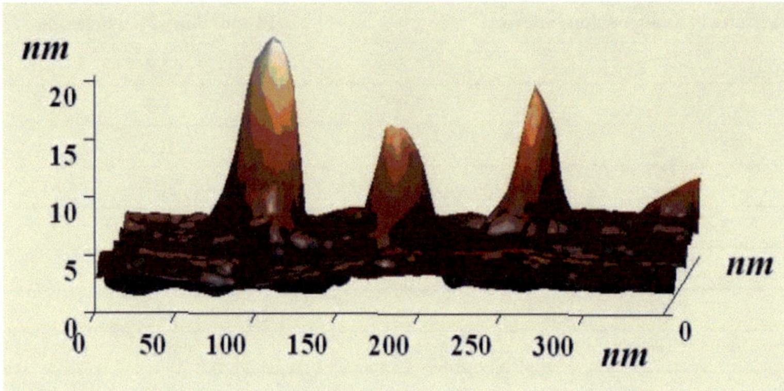

Figure 2.
The 3D-pattern of the MnO_2 nanodisperse particles, atomic force microscopy with the use of solver-PRO microscope (NT-MDT, Russian) [10].

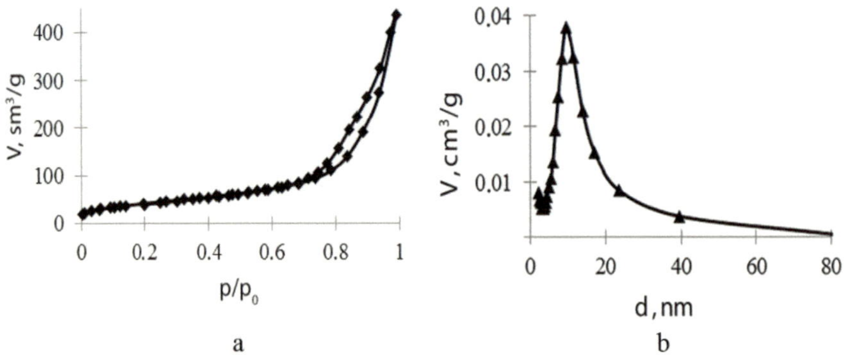

Figure 3.
Nanodisperse MnO_2: (a) nitrogen isotherm adsorption-desorption and (b) pore size distribution d (nm) [15].

covering graphite rods via electrochemical deposition, up-to-date sorbents with the use of vacuum-ultrasound laser ablation [17, 18]. Inhalation exposure of workers to nanosized MnO_2 particles is quite possible during such manufacturing processes as these particles are emitted into working area air. In relation to that, wider utilization of nanosized MnO_2 in industrial production as well as providing workers' safety in the process requires more profound studies on toxicity of nanodisperse MnO_2 when it enters a body being inhaled as an aerosol.

The authors used water suspension of nanodisperse MnO_2 in concentration equal to 36.0 ± 2.3 mg/cm^3 as an examined substance. To make comparison, microdisperse MnO_2 with concentration in manganese water suspension equal to 40.31 ± 1.6 mg/cm^3 was used. The particles size amounted to 5.5–37.0 μm (particles' share 67.0%). The size of microdisperse MnO_2 particles is 194–1300 times greater than the nanodisperse MnO_2 particles size. Specific surface area of MnO_2 nanoparticles (Brunauer-Emmett-Teller technique [13]) was equal to 150.23 m^2/g, which was 1.2 times higher than microparticle-specific surface area (130 m^2/g). This property can cause high MnO_2 nanoparticles reactivity *in vitro* and *in vivo* [19].

To determine acute toxicity parameters, the authors completed an experiment on pubescent Wistar rats (male and female) with body weight equal to 190 ± 10 g. They examined and assessed acute toxicity of nanodisperse MnO_2 water suspension at inhalation introduction as an aerosol in accordance with Interstate Standard "Testing techniques on determining chemical products effects exerted on a human body: acute inhalation toxicity technique determining acute toxicity class

(ATC technique)" (OECD, Test No 436:2008, IDT) (2012). Inhalation introduction into the experimental animals' bodies was modeled in inhalation system with integrated software; and a chamber for a whole body was used in the process (TSE Systems GmbH, Germany). The experimental animals were divided into three groups (experimental groups were 1 and 2, and group 3 was a control one, n = 18 animals). Experimental group 1 was exposed to the examined substance inhalation at substance nominal concentration in the chamber equal to 0.05 mg/l; concentration for experimental group 2 was equal to 0.5 mg/l. The exposure lasted for 4 hours; the animals received no nutrition during the process. After inhalation exposure, the animals were observed during next 96 hours to detect possible delayed substance toxicity. Control group was exposed to inhalation of distilled water in the form of an aerosol under analogous conditions. The water conformed to TU 6-09-2502-77. After observation period for the animals from experimental groups 1 and 2 was over, they were taken out of the experiment via sparing euthanasia. Brains were extracted with a special instrument and fixed in 5% solution of buffered neutral formalin. Fixed tissue pieces were dehydrated in Excelsior ES automatic histological processor (Thermo Scientific, Germany). The finished specimens were examined in Axio Lab A1 light-optical microscope, micropictures were taken with the use of Mikroskopkamera AxioCam ERc 5 s (Carl Zeiss, Germany) at magnification equal to ×400.

The results of all research performed with independent techniques application helped to detect that the examined MnO_2 sample was a nanomaterial. The examination of the tested substance suspension in concentration equal to 36.0 ± 2.3 mg/cm^3 proves it. Particle size distribution on the bar graph is as follows (particles cross-section size is presented): 13 nm (1.2% of the total particles number), 15–29 nm (94.4%), and 33–100 nm (4.1%). Maximum peak of particles size corresponded to 19 ± 4 nm (41.2%). Scanning electron microscopy technique enabled detecting that visualized particles size exceeded 20 nm. Assessment of nanoparticles quantity in the inhalation chamber area showed that when nanodisperse fraction is fed into the chamber and transfers into aerosol, it does not agglomerate to micrometer range (**Figures 4** and **5**). The size of most particles (99% from the total quantity) does not exceed 100 nm at the examined actual concentrations after 2–4 hours of exposure.

Clinical picture of acute intoxication at inhalation exposure to nanodisperse MnO_2 aerosol at actual concentration equal to 0.029 ± 0.001 mg/dm^3 was characterized with evident neurotoxic effects, which started to occur in male and female rats from experimental group 1 after 3 hours of exposure. Animals had movement coordination disorders, took unusual postures, and showed weaker reaction to sound stimulus; all these effects remained in survivor animals during 48 hours after exposure. When actual concentration was equal to 0.472 ± 0.005 mg/dm^3, rats started to suffer from apparent respiratory failure after 30 minutes of exposure.

Most rats in experimental group 2 (three male and two female) died within 150–190 minutes after the experiment started; their death was caused by acute respiratory failure. One female rat died 2 hours after the experiment was over. The animals were sluggish before their death, they took lateral position, and demonstrated no reaction to sound stimulus or motion activity. Death of the experimental animals was not established. CL_{50} of the examined nanodisperse MnO_2 amounted to 0.12 mg/l. This concentration is within 0.05–0.5 mg/l range, which allows to define the tested substance as having the second hazard class "ATC technique" (OECD, Test No. 436:2008, IDT). It is known that minimal toxic concentration (TCL_0) of nanosized MnO_2 for rats at inhalation introduction during 24 hours amounts to 1.8 mg/m^3; for mice during 7 hours, 49 mg/m^3 (data taken from Minimal lethal dose (LDL_0) for rats at intratracheal introduction amount to 45 mg/kg. Safety specification does not contain any additional information regarding errors, confidence limits, or animals sex. Morphologic changes in brain tissues of the rats from

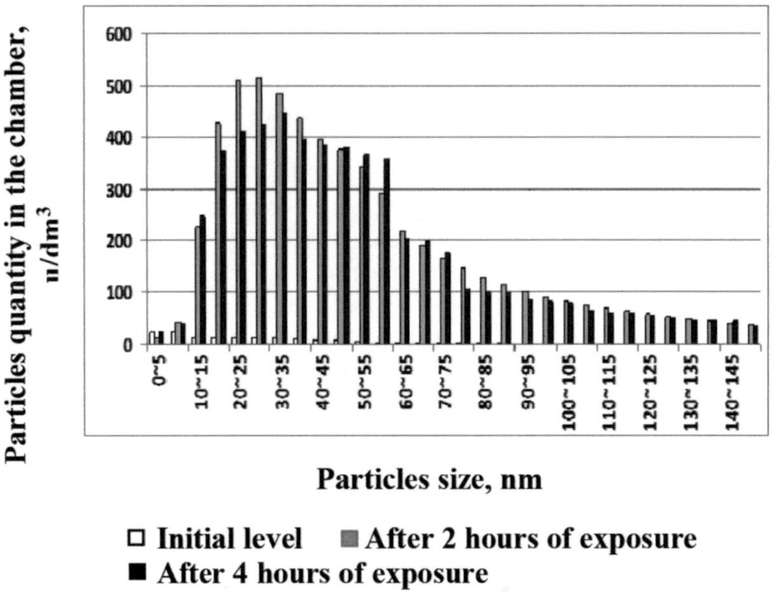

Figure 4.
Nanoparticle concentration in the inhalation chamber air at actual MnO_2 concentration equal to 0.029 ± 0.001 *mg/dm*^{3} *[15].*

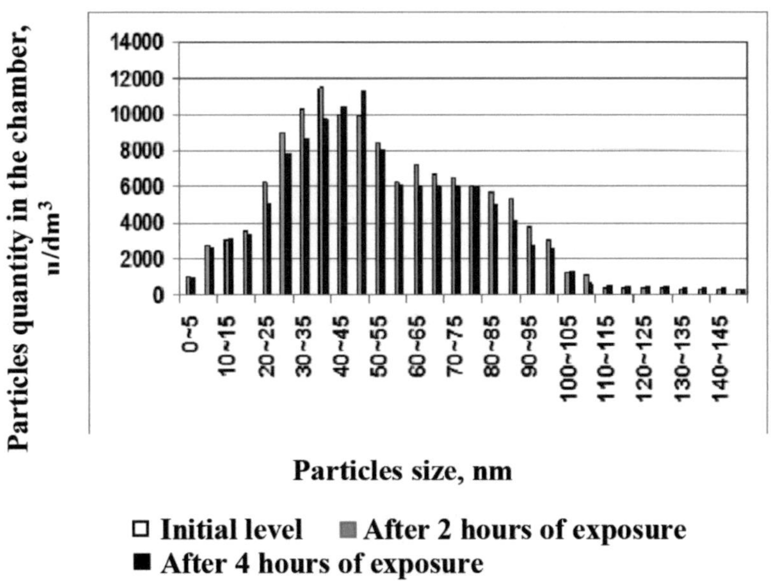

Figure 5.
Nanoparticle concentration in the inhalation chamber air at actual MnO_2 concentration equal to 0.472 ± 0.005 *mg/dm*^{3} *[15].*

experimental group 1 in comparison with control group were characterized with the following pathologic disorders: brain substance vessels were filled with blood insignificantly or moderately and had focal endothelium swelling and perivascular spaces dilatation. The most apparent changes in brain tissue of the rats from experimental group 1 occurred in cerebellum. Neurons and neuroglia cells were characterized with grave ischemic damages in the form of wrinkling and pyknosis. Nerve fibers of brain tissue looked spongy and were unevenly colored, had fizzy contours, and focal prolapse of glial elements (**Figure 6**).

The results obtained in the course of the research indicate that the examined nanosized MnO_2 particles can cause neurotoxic effect and respiratory failure; the combination of these two factors could lead to the animals' death. The obtained results are confirmed by research performed by a number of authors [20, 21], which prove that MnO_2 nanoparticles exert toxic effects at inhalation exposure. Thus, after 24-hour exposure, catalytic generation of active oxygen forms (AOF) in human alveolar epithelial cells [20] increased; level of extracellular and intracellular oxidized glutathione form (GSSG) also grew by 30 and 80% correspondingly [20, 21]. Manganese oxide (IV) nanoparticles sized up to 30 nm are able to penetrate into neuron-like PC-12 cells of a brain at inhalation exposure via olfactory nerve [22] and accumulate in astrocytes [17, 23].

Here, slight mitochondrial activity inhibition occurs; dose-dependent decrease in dopamine and its metabolites (3,4-dihydroxyphenylacetic acid and homovanillic acid) takes place. This process is accompanied with a multiple AOF growth [20, 24] and becomes apparent in experimental animals through neurodegenerating disorders as early as after 2 or 3 weeks of exposure [20, 23, 24]. It is proved that MnO_2 nanoparticles (III, IV) can accumulate in brain cells [25, 26]. In particular, astrocytes are able to accumulate MnO_2 nanoparticles and produce AOF [25, 27, 28]. This process is accompanied with protein cleavage activation mediated by caspase-3 and protein kinase Cδ (these are enzymes that participate in apoptosis, necrosis, and inflammatory processes), as well as phosphorylation cycle activation [25, 26]. As particles concentration increases, level of p38 mutagen-active protein kinase grows linearly; this protein kinase activates apoptotic mechanism of untimely cell death [24, 29–31]. Tumor necrosis factor-α doubles in olfactory bulb, frontal cortex, midbrain, and striate body [27]. If inhalation exposure to MnO_2 nanoparticles (III, IV) is long-term, time-depending activation of transferrin in dopaminergic nervous cells is detected, as well as structural changes in Beclin 1 and LC3 proteins, which, in its turn, can be an evidence of potential autophagia process activation [20].

As per data taken from the annotated scientific literature, it is proved that toxic effects exerted on nervous system cells can be caused both by nanoparticles [25, 29] and by microdisperse analog at a low-dose exposure [32]. Disorders in neurons membranes functions can underlie the neurotoxic action mechanism; such disorders result from membranes lipid peroxidation which in its turn is caused by direct cytotoxic effect of nanoparticles determined for dopaminergic

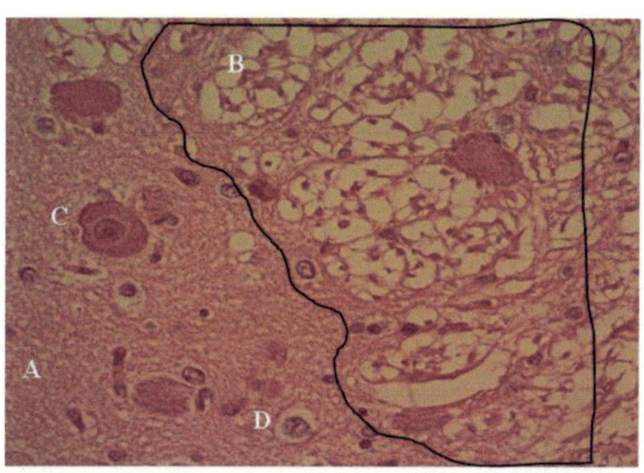

Figure 6.
Cerebellum of a Wistar rat after acute inhalation exposure to nanodisperse MnO_2 aerosol at actual MnO_2 concentration in the inhalation chamber area equal to 0.029 ± 0.001 mg/dm³ (painted with hematoxylin-eosin, ×400): A is cerebellum tissue without changes, green; B is ischemia focus (grave ischemic changes), edema (damage zone is outlined); C is motor neuron of cerebellum subcortex; and D is glia cells with pericellular space dilatation [15].

neurons [25, 29, 33]. This effect can be more apparent for nanodisperse particles in comparison with microdisperse analog effects due to the fact that nanoparticles have a greater specific surface area.

Mechanism of nanodisperse MnO_2 neurotoxicity is related to the ability to generate free radicals and to interact with proteins. Manganese oxide nanoparticles are able to actively generate free radicals when they interact with bilipid layer of cell membranes [25, 30]. When interacting with cell membranes, they stimulate excessive creation of active oxygen forms (AOF), which is accompanied with high catalytic activity and cell apoptosis [25, 26, 30]. Oxidized (GSSG) and reduced glutathione form (GSH) content is one of the parameters showing oxidative stress level. It is proved that if alveolar epithelial cells are exposed to MnO_2 particles for 24 hours, the level of extracellular and intracellular GSSG increases by 30 and 80% correspondingly; at the same time, caspase-3 activity grows and this enzyme is known to induce apoptosis processes. GSH concentration increases after 24-hour exposure to the examined substance, and it can be caused by activation of γ-glutamylcysteine synthetase synthesis and more active feed system of cystine and glutamate amino acids, which are substrates for synthesis of reduced glutathione form [25]. A significant increase in GSSG in a cell induced by MnO_2 nanoparticles can be caused by manganese particles entering reduction reaction with superoxide formation, which, under superoxide dismutase effects, is converted into oxygen and hydrogen peroxide. Then, hydrogen peroxide decomposes with the help of reduced glutathione form, and it leads to GSSG increase. Another possible way of hydrogen peroxide transformation in a cell is hydroxyl radicals creation in the presence of manganese ions; these radicals are also able to oxidize GSH with creation of GSSG [26].

Clinical picture of acute intoxication, detailed in the previous works by the authors [34], confirms the mechanism of toxic effects exerted by nanodisperse MnO_2 particles which a number of authors describe in above-mentioned scientific works [27, 28]. Respiratory failure evolvement can also be related to potential ability of the examined nanoparticles to cause inflammatory changes with consequent apoptosis of alveolar epithelial cells. At the same time, MnO_2 nanoparticles have greater resistance to mucociliary clearance; therefore, they are in a longer contact with respiratory tract cells in comparison with microdisperse analog [28].

3.2.2 Examination of acute toxicity which nanodisperse MnO_2 has at oral introduction

Intensive development of the major promising nanotechnological spheres such as nano-optics, nanoelectronics, pharmacology, chemistry, and metallurgy has direct influence on growth of nanodisperse MnO_2 production volumes. Nanosized MnO_2 particles are widely used in production of matrixes for nanomagnetic materials and sorbents [35], nanoaccelerators, semiconductor thermistors [36]. Wastes of such productions can get into sewage and then into water reservoirs serving as sources for drinking water supply. MnO_2 nanoparticles are known to have nonspherical form, which makes for lower speed of their excretion out of a body with the help of immune system's phagocytes through lymphatic ducts and causes their longer contacts with body tissues [19]. In relation to that it is reasonable to think that profound examination of nanodisperse MnO_2 aerosol toxicity at oral introduction with water into a body is of great importance for securing production workers safety and safety of population living in areas influenced by such productions.

The authors examined nanodisperse MnO_2 water suspension with particles sized 15–29 nm. Particles were thread-like and had surface area equal to $150.2 \pm 2.6\ m^2/g$. MnO_2 concentration in nanodisperse solution was equal to $36.0 \pm 2.3\ mg/cm^3$.

The detailed description of synthesis and physical and chemical properties of nanodisperse MnO_2 is given in the precious works [37, 38]. To make comparison, microdisperse MnO_2 with concentration in manganese water suspension equal to 40.31 ± 1.6 mg/cm^3 was used. The particle size amounted to 5.5–37.0 μm (particles' share 67.0%) (dynamic light scattering technique with the use of Microtrac S3500 laser analyzer (Microtrac, the USA)). The size of microdisperse MnO_2 particles is 194–1300 times greater than nanodisperse MnO_2 particle size. Specific surface area of MnO_2 nanoparticles (Brunauer–Emmett–Teller technique [13]) was equal to 150.23 m^2/g, which was 1.2 times higher than microparticles specific surface area (130 m^2/g). Acute toxicity parameters of nanodisperse MnO_2 were assessed as per the results of comprehensive acute experiments performed in accordance with methodical guidelines [10] on nonlinear male white mice with body weight equal to 27 ± 2 г (M ± m) (n = 70); the animals belonged to a conventional category. Nanodisperse MnO_2 was introduced into mice's bodies a single time via gastric tube in various doses: group 1 received 2000 mg/kg of body weight, group 2–3500 mg/kg, and group 3–5000 mg/kg. The tested sample was introduced in a form of water suspension in volume equal to 1–2% of the animals' body weight. Microdisperse MnO_2 was introduced into mice from experimental groups 4, 5, and 6 in the same doses as in groups 1, 2, and 3. The tested samples were introduced in the same way. Control group 7 received water a single time via gastric tube in the same volume. The observation term after the tested substances was introduced amounted to 14 days. Mice were kept in cages: five animals in each.

The experiment revealed that clinical picture of acute intoxication at introducing nano- and microdisperse MnO_2 solutions is uniform and nonspecific. Animals from experimental groups 1–6 suffered from hyperexcitability and convulsions during the first 20 minutes of the experiment; then inhibition state occurred, animals' reaction to sound and pain became weak, they had hypopnoe. Animals in experimental groups 2 and 3 died mostly during the first 24 hours; in group 1, during 48 hours; and in comparison groups 5 and 6 in the period from 48 to 72 hours. No mice from group 4 or 7 died in the course of the experiment. It was detected that if nanodisperse MnO_2 solution was once introduced into a body via gastric tube, LD_{50} amounted to 2340 ± 602.6 mg/kg of body weight (third hazard class); in case of microdisperse MnO_2 solution introduction, the dose was equal to 6000 ± 485.6 mg/kg (fourth hazard class). Average death time (TL_{50}) for mice after intragastric introduction of nanodisperse MnO_2 solution amounted to 35.2 hours. When microdisperse MnO_2 solution was introduced, TL_{50} amounted to 32 hours. Cumulation index amounted to 0.79 for nanodisperse MnO_2 particles. If cumulation index is >5, one can assume that nanoparticles are hypercumulative. Cumulation index is equal to 0 for microdisperse MnO_2 particles. If cumulation index is equal to 0, one can assume that particles are moderately cumulative [39].

Analysis of changes, which occurred in venous blood of the experimental animals, revealed that nanoparticles of disperse MnO_2 solution in a dose equal to 3500 and 5000 mg/kg exert more apparent toxic effects on erythrocytes and thrombocytes in comparison with a microdisperse analog. It is confirmed by polychromatocytes occurrence as their share amounted to 20 and 35% of the total erythrocytes number in peripheral blood of mice from experimental groups 2 and 3 correspondingly. When microdisperse MnO_2 was introduced in the same doses polychromatocytes share in mice's blood amounted to 10 and 15% correspondingly. 10–20% of erythrocytes in blood of mice from those groups contained pathologic Jolly bodies and it was two times higher than the same parameter in blood of mice from experimental groups 5 and 6 correspondingly. Nanodisperse MnO_2 solution caused massive thrombocytes aggregation in blood of mice from experimental groups 2 and 3. Microdisperse MnO_2 solution when introduced into mice in a dose equal to 5000 mg/kg (experimental group 6) led to only sporadic occurrence of thrombocytes aggregation. There were no pathologic changes in blood slides of mice from experimental group 7.

Morphological examinations after introducing nanodisperse MnO_2 solution in a dose equal to 3500 mg/kg revealed changes in all examined organs taken out of mice. There was significant dilatation and hyperemia of veins in liver and kidneys, considerable blood overflow in veins of cardiac muscle and epicardium, as well as in heart chambers. There were hemorrhages detected in medullar substance of kidneys. Proliferative processes occurred in macrophage and lymphoid systems of experimental animals. An increased number of macrophages and their activation was detected in liver, in both kidneys and, in particular, in lungs (**Figure 7**). Kupffer cells in liver are enlarged and bulged into sinusoid capillaries lumen; mesangial cells in renal bodies are hypertrophic, and numerous alveolar macrophages contain phagocyte material. Lymphoid nodules in spleen white pulp are enlarged, tend to fuse, and there is no typical division into zones in them. Red pulp prevails in the organ together with diffuse and focal lymphatization occurrence. Proliferation of cells from lymphocytes and macrophages range leads to leukocytic infiltration of parenchymatous organs. Numerous periportal and intralobular lymphoid-histiocytic infiltrates occur in liver; perivascular and intertubular ones are observed in kidneys. Organ infiltration with lymphocytes is so active that it can penetrate through blood-brain barrier; lymphoid infiltrates can be detected even in white substance of cerebral hemispheres (**Figures 8–10**).

When a microdisperse MnO_2 solution in a dose equal to 3500 mg/kg was introduced, it led to some dilatation of sinusoid capillaries in liver and vessels of renal microcirculatory bed. Capsule lumen in some renal corpuscles was dilated. Occasional lymph-histiocytic infiltration occurred in parenchymatous organs. Infiltrates were located only in connective tissue and were rather small. As opposed to group 2, animals from group 5 had no infiltrates in brain hemispheres cortex. There was only slight perivascular and moderate pericellular edema located mostly in granular layer.

Therefore, mice from group 2 after a single introduction of nanodisperse MnO_2 solution in a dose equal to 3500 mg/kg via gastric tube had more apparent morphological changes in internal organs than mice from group 5 (microdisperse analog). These changes were detected in circulatory system and characterized with dilatation and hyperemia of veins in all the studied organs. Blood overflow in veins of cardiac

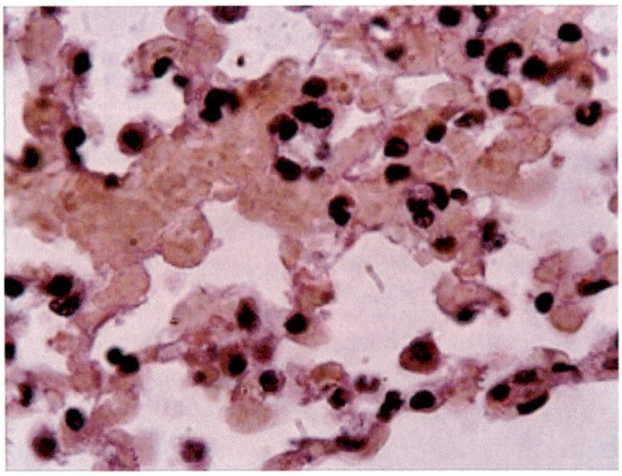

Figure 7.
Macrophage reaction in a lung of a mouse from experimental group 2, which died during the first day after nanodisperse MnO_2 in a dose equal to 3500 mg/kg, was introduced. The specimen was painted with hematoxylin and eosin, and the magnification was equal to ×1000 [38].

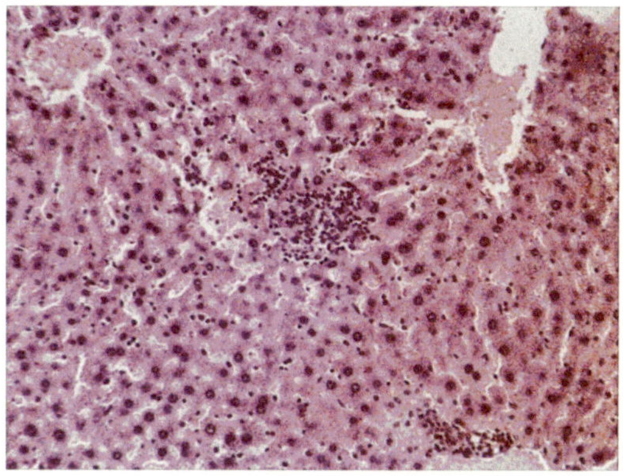

Figure 8.
A nonlinear mouse from experimental group 2, which died during the first day after nanodisperse MnO_2 in a dose equal to 3500 mg/kg, was introduced. Lymph-histiocytic intralobular infiltrates in a liver. The specimen is painted with hematoxylin and eosin, and magnification is equal to ×200 [38].

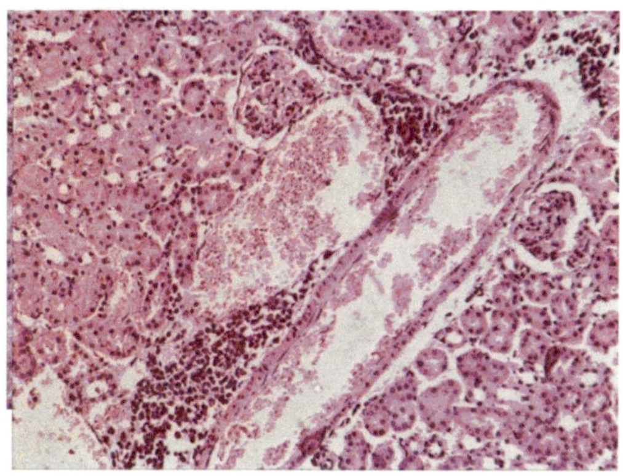

Figure 9.
A nonlinear mouse from experimental group 2, which died during the first day after nanodisperse MnO_2 in a dose equal to 3500 mg/kg, was introduced. Lymph-histiocytic perivascular infiltrates in a kidney. The specimen is painted with hematoxylin and eosin, and magnification is equal to ×200 [38].

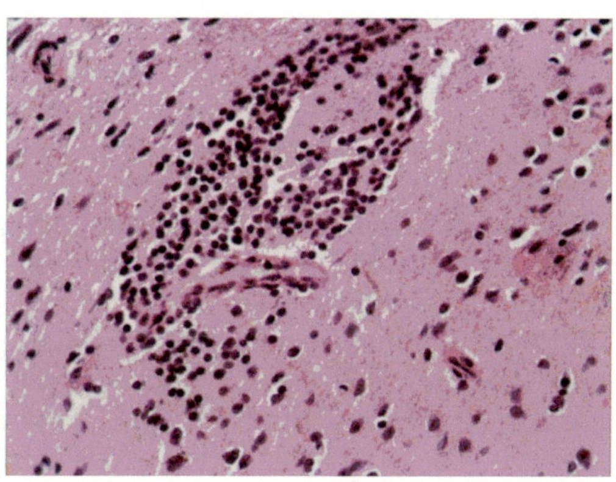

Figure 10.
A nonlinear mouse from experimental group 2, which died during the first day after nanodisperse MnO_2 in a dose equal to 3500 mg/kg, was introduced. The specimen is painted with hematoxylin and eosin, and magnification is equal to ×400. Lymphocytic infiltration in white substance of cerebral hemispheres [38].

muscle, epicardium and all heart chambers was particularly evident. Mice from group 5 had no peculiar morphological changes in circulatory system organs. Mice from group 2 had proliferative processes in lymphoid and macrophage systems. These processes were morphologically apparent through hypertrophy of thymus lobules cortex, lymphoid follicles of spleen white pulp and lymphatization of spleen red pulp, and macrophage activation in liver, kidneys and lungs. Such morphological changes did not occur in mice from group 5. Proliferation of lymphoid cells and macrophages leads to histioleukocytic infiltration of parenchymatous organs. And here, processes caused by nanodisperse MnO_2 solution impact are more apparent than those caused by microdisperse MnO_2 solution. Morphological changes are determined by vascular disorders in venous bed, which result in hemorrhages in parenchymatous organs, especially in kidneys. There were none of such morphological changes in mice when microdisperse MnO_2 solution was introduced into them. The analysis of the obtained results allows to make a conclusion that nanodisperse MnO_2 solution at a single introduction via gastric tube has LD_{50} equal to 2340 ± 602.6 mg/kg (third hazard class), which is 2.6 times higher than LD_{50} equal to 6000 ± 485.6 mg/kg at a single introduction of microdisperse MnO_2 solution (fourth hazard class). Nanodisperse MnO_2 solution at single introduction into mice via gastric tube in a dose equal to 3500 mg/kg exerts hemotoxic effects, which reveal themselves in a form of pathologic inclusions in erythrocytes and increased thrombocytes aggregation. There were also certain circulation disorders observed such as vein dilatation and hyperemia, as well as filling of their lumen with erythrocytes, which leads to hemorrhages in all the studied organs. Proliferative processes in lymphoid and macrophage systems were detected; they result in hypertrophy of thymus lobule cortex and lymphoid follicles of spleen white pulp, lymphatization of spleen red pulp, and macrophages activation in liver, kidneys and lungs.

3.3 Studying subchronic and chronic toxicity of nanodisperse manganese oxide water suspension at intragastric introduction via gastric tube

Studying subchronic toxicity of nanodisperse MnO_2 water suspension at intragastric introduction via gastric tube: nowadays, there is a growing interest in using MnO_2 nanoparticles as a sorbent and catalyst for complex purification of liquid radioactive wastes, which are dangerous for human health. But MnO_2 nanoparticles can get into sewage in the process and later they can be found in surface water reservoirs used for drinking water supply to population. In relation to that, study of toxic effects exerted by MnO_2 nanoparticles at oral introduction with drinking water matters a lot if one wants to assess their safety.

Experimental research dedicated to nanodisperse MnO_2 were performed with intragastric introduction via gastric tube during 90 days. During this particular research, nanodisperse MnO_2 water suspension was introduced into Wistar rats (males and females) with body weight equal to 200 ± 10 g (n = 100) via gastric tube daily for 90 days. Animals were divided into four experimental groups and 1 control group, 20 animals in each. Nanodisperse MnO_2 water suspension was introduced in the following doses: group 1—257.7 mg/kg (1/10 LD_{50}), group 2—51.54 mg/kg (1/50 LD_{50}), group 3—10.3 mg/kg (1/250 LD_{50}[3]), group 4—5.15 mg/kg (1/500 LD_{50}), and group 5 (control one)—distilled water in volume equal. Nanodisperse MnO_2 water suspension dispersion was accomplished directly before carrying out the research and later on a weekly basis during 90 days, while the experiment was lasting in order to achieve even particles distribution in a volume of liquid; the procedure was done with the use of ultrasound at room temperature under continuous pulsation at 65%-power for 2 minutes. The following parameters were assessed: body weight dynamics, as well as changes in biochemical parameters of neurons functions and oxidation-antioxidant system balance. Morphological changes in brain tissues were studied via histological specimens microscopy (magnification ×400).

Body weight dynamics analysis performed on rats from group 1 revealed authentic decrease in this parameter by 7.7% by the 30th day of the experiment in comparison with the baseline. Body weight was recovered by the 90th day. Decrease in body weight of rats from group 1 authentically differed from this parameter in control group during the whole experiment. In all other groups, authentic increase in body weight of experimental animals was detected. Examination and assessment of biochemical parameters characterizing neurotransmitters balance and oxidation-antioxidant system at long-term introduction of nanodisperse MnO_2 water suspension proves negative effects occurrence; these effects are dose depending. There was an authentic increase in lipid hydroperoxide level in blood serum of rats on the 30th day of the experiment when doses were 10.0–260 mg/kg of body weight; this parameter was 1.4–1.9 times higher than the baseline in rats from the control group ($p < 0.001$). Malonic dialdehyde level in blood serum of rats was 1.6–2.0 times higher than the baseline of this parameter in control group rats, the doses being equal ($p < 0.001$). On the 90th day, high levels of lipids hydroperoxides and malonic dialdehyde in blood serum remained. The order of discrepancy between the baseline and parameters in the control group was 1.3–1.9 times ($p < 0.001$). When a dose was equal to 5.0 mg/kg, there were not any authentic discrepancies between these parameters and the baseline, or between them and control group parameters during the whole experiment. When doses were 10.0–260 mg/kg, an authentic decrease in Cu/Zn-SOD and OAS in blood serum of rats was registered; this decrease was dose dependent. During the whole experiment, Cu/Zn-SOD level was on average from 1.4 to 4.6 times lower than the baseline and the control group parameter ($p < 0.001–0.002$). OAS level was 1.6–5.4 times lower ($p < 0.001$). When a dose was equal to 5.0 mg/kg, there were no authentic discrepancies in OAS level between experimental and control group during the whole experiment.

Assessment of basic neurotransmitters content in blood serum of rats on the 90th day of the experiment revealed authentic increase in glutamate level and decrease in GABA level in comparison with the baseline and control group. Changes in these parameters were dose dependent. Glutamate level in blood serum grew from 2 to 3.8 times depending on a dose ($p < 0.001$). GABA level in blood serum decreased 2.3–2.7 times ($p < 0.001$). When a dose was equal to 5.0 mg/kg, there was no authentic decrease in the analyzed parameters in blood serum against control group parameters. The obtained results show that, given their small size and high penetrability, MnO_2 nanoparticles can penetrate through blood-brain barrier and cause morphological-functional disorders in various sections of central nervous system when introduced into a body in different ways even in relatively small concentrations [27].

The detected activation of cell membranes lipid peroxidation and imbalance in CNS neuromediators at intragastric introduction of nanodispersed MnO_2, in Wistar rats, are confirmed by the results obtained by a number of authors at other ways of introduction into a body (for example, at intranasal, intratracheal, and inhalation introduction). As a number of authors state, when MnO_2 particle dose equals to 2.63 mg/kg and intranasal introduction of this dose lasts for 6 weeks, neurotoxicity can be observed as relative refractory period of a tail nerve grows [27]. Intratracheal introduction of MnO_2 nanoparticles in a dose equal to 2.63 mg/kg during 6 weeks leads to significant decrease in body weight, longer absolute refractory period of a tail nerve, and lower animals movability [27]. Neurotoxicity of MnO_2 nanoparticles at intratracheal introduction in doses equal to 2.63 and 5.26 mg/kg can be seen through increase in latent period of cortical potential occurrence (total response of large cortex neurons populations to synchronous impulses flow coming to them and caused by afferent irritator) in visual, auditory, and the first somatosensory area. This effect can be determined by disorders in neuron membranes functions as a result of membrane lipid peroxidation accompanied with calcium homeostasis disorders [23]. Nanoparticles and microparticles of MnO_2 in concentration equal to 100 μg/kg in saline were injected into rats once a 2 weeks during 14 weeks, and it allowed to determine that both substances caused authentic increase in dextrose and cholesterol level. MnO_2 nanoparticles lowered the level of high-density lipoproteins at the sixth, twelfth, and fourteenth week, while microdisperse analog caused such decrease at the twelfth week only. Researchers detected no authentic changes in triglyceride concentration. Changes in biochemical profile might be caused by oxidizing possibilities, which MnO_2 nanoparticles have [40]. An injection of MnO_2 nanoparticles into a rat's brain (in substantia nigra and tegmentum ventral area) in concentration equal to 87 μg/μl in 1 μl causes changes in locomotor abilities and spatial memory, which are related to dopaminergic neuron disorders and inflammation caused by nanoparticles. MnO_2 nanoparticles lead to early symptoms of extrapyramidal disorders with selective loss of dopaminergic neurons [27].

Histological specimens made of experimental animals' brains were assessed; the assessment results allowed to detect morphologic changes in tissue structure depending on a dose of nanodisperse MnO_2 water suspension. After a dose equal to 260 mg/kg of body weight a day had been introduced, the authors detected substantial vessels hyperemia in brain hemispheres cortex and cerebellum together with erythrocytes diapedesis and formation of subarachnoid hemorrhages focuses. There was also brain edema with perivascular and pericellular spaces dilatation (**Figure 11**). Focuses of nerve fibers demyelinization were detected as white substance fibers were unevenly painted and lighter areas with fizzy contours occurred.

After a 50 mg/kg dose focal perivascular and pericellular spaces dilatations form in brain cortex layers, but cortex layers still remain differentiated (**Figure 12**). Vessels in brain cortex tissues substance have thin walls, are moderately filled with blood, the endothelium is flattened, and there are small focal subarachnoid hemorrhages and focal neurons dystrophy zones. A slight perivascular spaces dilatation occurred after a 10 mg/kg of body weight a day (**Figure 13**). But when a dose was equal to 5 mg/kg of body weight a day, morphologic picture of brain and cerebellum tissues corresponded to that of control group; structure patterns were preserved in all the sections (**Figure 14**).

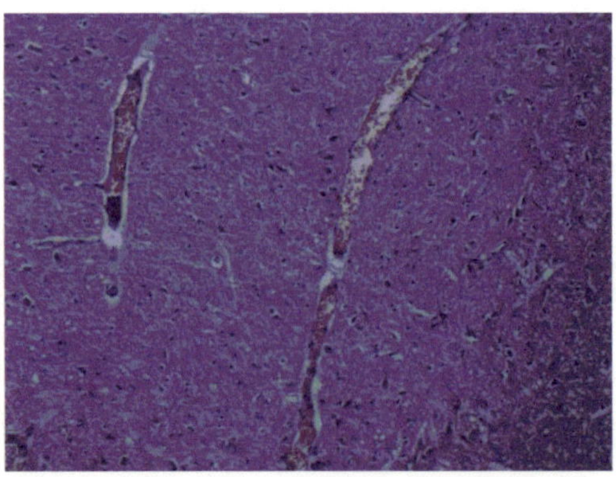

Figure 11.
Brain hemispheres cortex of a rat at intragastric introduction of nanodisperse MnO_2 water suspension in a dose equal to 260 mg/kg of body weight a day, 90th day of the experiment. There are dilated perivascular and pericellular spaces in brain cortex layers. Painted with hematoxylin and eosin, magnification ×400 [41].

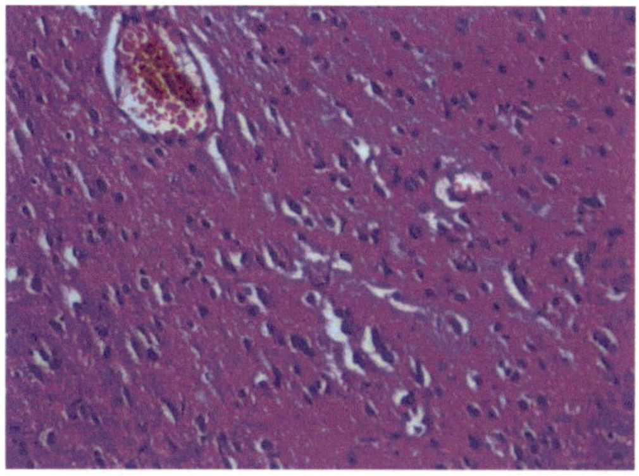

Figure 12.
Brain hemispheres cortex of a rat at intragastric introduction of nanodisperse MnO_2 water suspension in a dose equal to 50 mg/kg of body weight a day, 90th day of the experiment. There are dilated perivascular and pericellular spaces in brain cortex layers. Painted with hematoxylin and eosin, magnification ×400 [41].

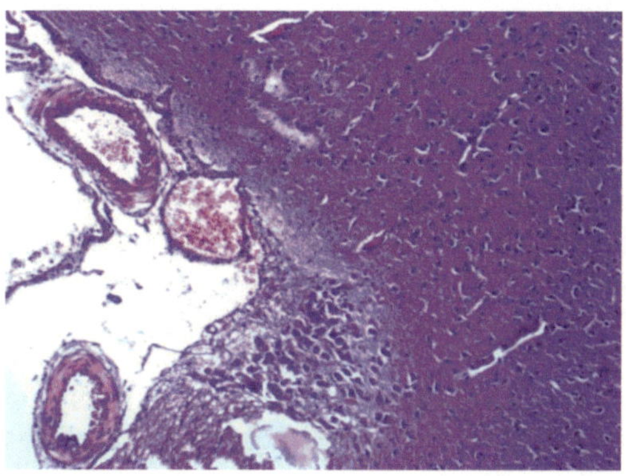

Figure 13.
Brain hemispheres cortex of a rat at intragastric introduction of nanodisperse MnO_2 water suspension in a dose equal to 10 mg/kg of body weight a day, 90th day of the experiment. There is slight perivascular spaces dilatation in brain hemispheres cortex. painted with hematoxylin and eosin, magnification ×100 [41].

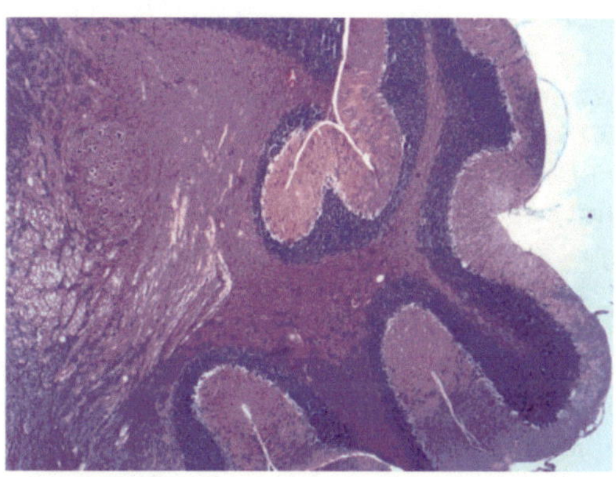

Figure 14.
Cerebellum of a rat at intragastric introduction of nanodisperse MnO_2 water suspension in a dose equal to 5 mg/kg of body weight a day, 90th day of the experiment. Tissue structure pattern in all cerebellum sections is preserved and corresponds to that of control group. Painted with hematoxylin and eosin, magnification ×100 [41].

Brain cortex tissues layers are differentiated quite well. External granular layer is formed out of solid bunch consisting of numerous small neurons; pyramidal layer of brain cortex is wide and consists of polymorphous neurons. Internal granular layer of brain cortex and cerebellum is thin, noncontinuous, made of small pyramidal and stellate cells; ganglionic layer cells in brain cortex tissues are large, polymorphous with dark nucleuses, diffusely located; there is a great number of diverse neurons (they differ in form and size) in polymorphous cells layer. Ganglionic layer in cerebellum tissue has one raw of Purkinje cells with well-developed eosinophilic granular cytoplasm and rounded dark nucleuses. Molecular layer in cerebellum tissue is spongy and contains a small number of minor cells. White substance in brain and cerebellum tissue is made of evenly painted nerve fibers bunches and rounded glia cells. Brain vessels have thin walls and are feebly or moderately filled with blood.

Comparison of pathomorphologic effects occurring at intragastric introduction of nanodisperse MnO_2 water suspension and microdisperse MnO_2 water suspension in a dose equal to 10 mg/kg during 90 days showed that pathomorphologic changes in brain and cerebellum tissues were much more apparent and wide-spread when nanodisperse MnO_2 was introduced. After introduction of nanodisperse MnO_2 water suspension more apparent changes occurred in circulatory system in a form of hemodynamic disorders with focal feeble and moderate vessels hyperemia in brain, liver, lungs, kidneys, and heart; there were also subarachnoid hemorrhages in brain. Changes in lymphatic system became evident through feeble and moderate perivascular lymph-macrophage infiltrates in lungs tissue penetrating into adjacent alveoli. Pathologic changes in macrophage system were apparent through alveolar macrophages activation with formation of small bunches in alveoli lumen. After introduction of microdisperse MnO_2 water suspension changes are represented by focal vessels hyperemia, subarachnoid hemorrhages in brain, small focal lymph-microphage infiltrates in lungs and gastrointestinal tract. Besides, after introduction of nanodisperse MnO_2 water suspension there was perivascular and pericellular spaces dilatation in brains, feebly apparent perivascular thin fibrous cardiosclerosis and feebly apparent focal protein dystrophy in hepatocytes; no such effects were detected after microdisperse MnO_2 introduction.

All the obtained materials were summarized; it allowed to make an assumption on a possible mechanism of toxic impact exerted by nanodisperse MnO_2 particles at oral introduction. Lipid peroxidation activation caused by direct damaging impact exerted by nanodisperse MnO_2 particles on bilipid layer of cytoplasmatic membrane can underlie the whole process [42]. High levels of lipid hydroperoxides and malonic dialdehyde in blood serum are the evidence of this effect. Lower levels of Cu/Zn-SOD and OAS in blood serum prove antioxidation processes insufficiency. The results obtained in the research showed that astrocytes and neurons membranes are the first targets influenced by nanodisperse MnO_2 water suspension at oral introduction, just as at inhalation one [21, 26]. In case of oral introduction it can be determined by apparent ability of nanodisperse MnO_2 particles to penetrate into blood from gastrointestinal tract. MnO_2 nanoparticles reach brain tissues coming from bloodstream through capillary endothelial cells of blood brain barrier and accumulate in astrocytes [26]. Damaged astrocytes due to enhanced peroxidation of cells membranes lipids and active oxygen forms occurrence can lose their ability to capture and neutralize excessive quantities of "exciting" amino acid, namely glutamate; thus, excitotoxic effect evolves [43]. It becomes apparent as glutamate concentration in blood serum grows and GABA content in it decreases.

Morphological changes in brain tissues prove pathogenetic impact exerted by MnO_2 nanoparticles which was detected in the process of biochemical parameters assessment. Degenerative changes evolvement can be caused by direct oxidative influence which nanoparticles have on neurons, glia cells, and vessels endothelium. The detected effects can only result from direct contact between nanoparticles and brain tissues which is the evidence of probable penetration through blood-brain barrier. The results of examining morphologic changes in brain tissues of Wistar rats, which were obtained at sub-acute intragastric introduction of nanodispersed MnO_2, enrich the existing data at sub-chronic intragastric introduction of MnO_2 nanoparticles, obtained by other authors. When MnO_2 nanoparticles are once a day introduced into rats' bodies orally during 28 days they are absorbed, accumulated in tissues after exposure and reveal their toxicity in doses lower than in case of micro-disperse analog [44].

Some authors present data showing that chronic effects exerted by MnO_2 nanoparticles lead to its accumulation in liver tissues with their consequent damage [45]. Histopathologic examinations revealed that MnO_2 nanoparticles had toxic influence on liver and kidneys [46]. There is an assumption that manganese is transported to organs with significant mitochondria content (to liver, pancreas and hypophysis in particular) where it is accumulated very fast [47].

Thus, the research revealed that nanodisperse MnO_2 water suspension, when being introduced daily into Wistar rats via gastric tube in doses equal to 260, 50, 10 mg/kg of body weight/a day during 90 days, causes lipid peroxidation activation (higher levels of lipid hydroperoxides and malonic dialdehyde in blood serum), and decrease in antioxidation system activity (lower OAS and Cu/Zn-SOD concentrations in blood serum). MnO_2 nanoparticles damage neurons and astrocytes membranes and lead to improper neurotransmitters ratio (higher glutamate concentration and lower GABA in blood serum). Pathomorphologic brain disorders occurred, such as vessels hyperemia, subarachnoid hemorrhages, brain edema with perivascular and pericellular spaces dilatation, focuses of nerve fibers demyelinization, focal dystrophic changes in vessels endothelium.

When a dose of nanodisperse MnO_2 water suspension was equal to 5 mg/kg of body weight/a day the substance did not exert any toxic effects.

Studying chronic toxicity of nanodisperse MnO_2 water suspension at intragastric introduction via gastric tube: toxicity of nanodisperse MnO_2 water suspension was examined at intragastric introduction via gastric tube under chronic experiment conditions; the examination was accomplished in full conformity with Methodical guidelines on toxicological-hygienic assessment of nanomaterial safety and Methodical guidelines on assessment order when assessing toxic effects exerted by nanomaterials on laboratory animals [48, 49].

To examine chronic toxicity of nanodisperse MnO_2 water suspension, a comprehensive experiment was performed on white male Wistar rats with body weight equal to 90 ± 5 g (n = 360). specific and integral parameters of negative effects in target organs were studied at daily intragastric introduction of nanodisperse MnO_2 water suspension via gastric tube. The experiment lasted for 180 days. The tested substance was daily introduced intragastrically via gastric tube, one time a day, the interval between introductions amounted to 24 hours. Mn concentration in water suspension in terms of MnO_2 was determined it amounted to 41.37 ± 2.5 mg/cm^3. Nanodisperse MnO_2 water suspension was introduced in the following doses: group 1–2.5 mg/kg (1/1000 LD_{50}); group 2–0.25 mg/kg (1/10,000 LD_{50}); group 3–0.05 mg/kg (1/50,000 $LD_{50}{}^3$); group 4 (control one)—distilled water in volume equal. The substance concentration in the suspension was controlled weekly. There were several assessments of animals' overall health state, their survival rate, and body weight dynamics; these assessments took place just before the experiment beginning, then on the 30th day, 60th day, 90th day, 120th day, 150th day, and 180th day of the experiment. Blood samples were taken from animals of all groups out of a caudal vein; biochemical and hematologic parameters were detected before the experiment beginning, on the 30th day and on the 180th day.

The authors selected parameters for assessing animals body responses at chronic introduction of the tested substance in accordance with Methodical guidelines on toxicological-hygienic assessment of nanomaterial safety [48]. Animals were taken out of the experiment on the 180th day via sparing euthanasia with carbon dioxide. After euthanasia they were autopsied, and microscopic assessment of morphological changes in internal organs followed. Nanodisperse MnO_2 particles were identified in blood of experimental animals at intragastric introduction via gastric tube on the 180th day of the experiment.

The obtained results revealed that hair state, motion activity, food consumption, and body weight of experimental animals in experimental groups did not have any discrepancies with the same parameters in the control group during the whole experiment. Body weight dynamics of animals from experimental groups did not differ authentically from body weight dynamics of animals from control group. There were no deaths of experimental animals in experiment and control groups at introduction of nanodisperse MnO_2water suspension during the whole observation period.

Basing on the analysis of changes in hematologic and biochemical blood parameters of Wistar rats from groups 1 and 2 against group 4, the following negative effects, which characterize toxicity of nanosized MnO_2 water suspension, were highlighted:

1. *Oxidizing-antioxidant balance:* lipid peroxidation activation was detected as per lipid hydroperoxide growth in blood serum and MDA growth in blood plasma. Lipid hydroperoxide concentration in blood serum of experimental animals grew on the 30th day of the experiment; it grew 2.5 times in group 1 and 1.6 times in group 2 in comparison with the same parameter in group 4. On the 180th day of the experiment, these parameters were 2.0 and 1.7 times higher in comparison with the group 4 ($p = 0.001–0.003$). Increased MDA content was detected in experimental animals from group 1 and 2 on the 30th day of the experiment, and it was 1.9 times higher than in group 4 ($p = 0.001–0.002$). This parameter was at the same level as in group 4 on the 180th day of the experiment. There was a decrease in antioxidation system activity. On the 30th day of the experiment, animals from group 1 had authentic 1.4 times lower activity of Cu/Zn-SOD than the same parameter in group 4. This parameter in animals from group 2 was 1.3 times lower than in group 4. On the 180th day of the experiment, Cu/Zn-SOD in animals from group 1 was 1.5 times lower; and in animals from group 2, 1.4 times lower ($p = 0.001–0.005$). Level of AOS in animals from group 1 was 4.7 times lower than in animals from group 4 on the 30th day of the experiment; the same parameter in group 2 was 5.9 times lower. On the 180th day, AOS in group 1 was 3.5 times lower; and in group 2, 4.1 times lower ($p = 0.001–0.002$). AOS and Cu/ZN-SOD parameters in group 3 corresponded to the same parameters in group 4 during the whole experiment.

2. *Neurotransmitter balance violation:* animals in group 1 had 1.4 times lower dopamine level in blood serum on the 30th day of the experiment; and animals in group 2, 1.7 times lower level than animals in group 4 ($p = 0.002$). On the 180th day of the experiment, dopamine decreased 1.7 times in group 1 and 1.9 times in group 2. By the 30th day of the experiment, there was an increase in glutamate level in blood serum in groups 1 and 2 in comparison with group 4; this parameter was 2.5 and 3.3 times higher correspondingly ($p = 0.0011$). By the 180th day of the experiment, glutamate level in group 1 was 1.9 times higher than in group 4 and 3.7 times higher in group 2 ($p = 0.001$). GABA level

in blood serum of animals from group 1 on the 20th day of the experiment was 1.3 times lower; and in group 2, 1.5 times lower than in group 4; this parameter in groups 1 and 2 was 2.2 times lower than in group 4 on the 180th day of the experiment ($p = 0.0011$). There were not any authentic changes in these parameters in animals from group 3.

3. *Inflammatory effect:* inflammatory effect was detected in groups 1 and 2 as per 1.6 times increase in CRP level on the 30th day of the experiment; on the 180th day, it was 1.9 times higher than in control group ($p = 0.001–0.002$). Animals from group 1 had higher TNF on the 30th day of the experiment (5.5 times higher), and animals from group 2, 6.8 times higher in comparison with the same parameter in group 4 ($p = 0.001$). On the 180th day of the experiment, TNF increased 4.4 times in group 1 and 5.4 times in group 2.

4. *Insufficiency of bowels brush border epithelium:* lower activity of β-galactosidase in blood serum may indicate that insufficiency of brush border epithelium in bowels evolves. This parameter was 3.9 times lower in group 1 and 2.9 times lower in group 2 in comparison with group 4 on the 180th day of the experiment ($p = 0.001$). There were not any changes in this parameter in group 3 against the control level.

5. *Electrolyte balance violation* electrolyte balance violation was detected in group 1 as there was an authentic decrease in K level in blood serum on the 180th day. The level was 1.3 times lower than the same parameter level in group 4 ($p = 0.011$).

6. *Sensitization:* sensitization occurrence was detected as per EO increase in blood on the 30th day of the experiment. It grew 1.8 times in group 1 and 1.9 times in group 2 in comparison with this parameter level in group 4 ($p = 0.013–0.026$). EO-LY level increased 1.3–1.7 times and 1.3 times against the control parameter ($p = 0.001–0.036$). MO level decreased 1.6 times in group 1 on the 30th day; later this parameter grew 1.5 times on the 180th day ($p = 0.006–0.023$). Sensitization in animals from groups 1 and 2 remained on the 180th day as MO quantity increased 1.4–1.45 times, NE quantity decreased 1.5–1.7 times, and EO quantity decreased 3.7–5.1 times against group 4 ($p = 0.001–0.016$). There were not any authentic changes in the examined parameters in group 3 in comparison with control group during the whole experiment. As the remaining biochemical parameters were assessed, no authentic discrepancies were revealed between experimental groups and control group.

No authentic changes in the examined parameters were detected against the control group when nanodisperse MnO_2 water suspension was introduced in a dose equal to 0.05 mg/kg during 180 days. Electronic microscopy of animals' whole blood did not reveal any nanodisperse particles in blood of animals from group 4. X-ray spectrometry analysis did not reveal any Mn particles either (**Figure 15**). When nanodisperse MnO_2 water suspension was introduced intragastrically via gastric tube into Wistar rates in a dose equal to 0.25 mg/kg (1/10,000 LD_{50}) during 180 days there were bunches of particles which were ellipsoid-shaped and needle-shaped on electronic images. There were not any such particles in blood of rats from the control group (**Figure 16**). The size of these particles lies within 90–130 nm range, and it can be determined by their agglomeration.

In spite of the fact that X-ray spectrometry analysis did not reveal any Mn content in blood of experimental animals, which received a dose equal to 0.25 mg/kg (and it can be due to spatial resolution inaccuracy of this technique), visualized particles were considered to be Mn nanosized particles as they are identical with the pure suspension sample of the tested substance and are not detected in blood of animals from the control group.

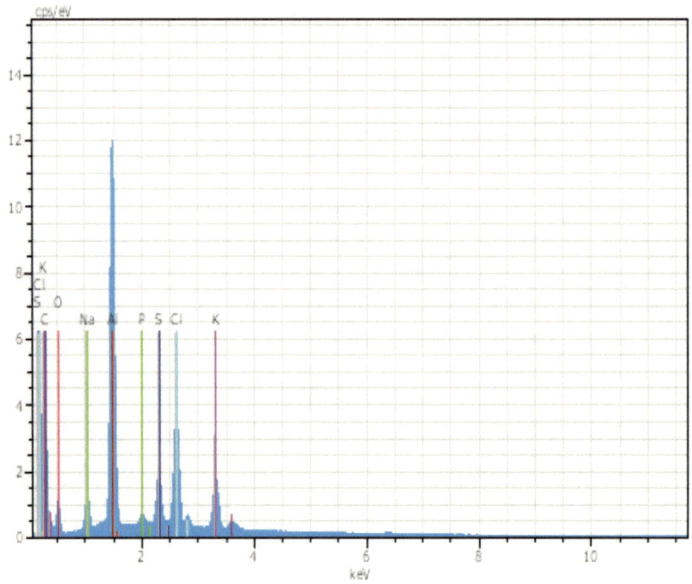

Figure 15.
X-ray spectrometry analysis of whole blood taken from a male Wistar rat form the control group [50].

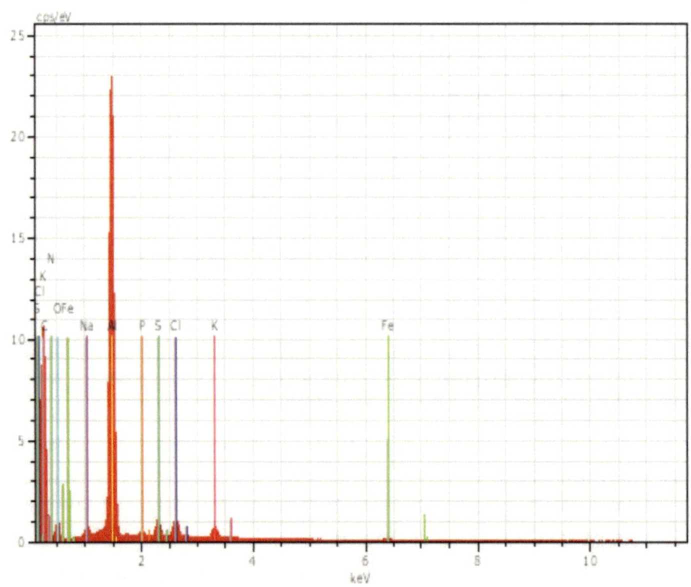

Figure 16.
X-ray spectrometry analysis of whole blood taken from an experimental animal, which received nanodisperse MnO_2 in a dose equal to 0.25 mg/kg [50].

4. Examining and assessing potential reproductive and mutagenic toxicity of nanodisperse manganese oxide water suspension at oral introduction with water

Embryotoxicity means capability of a chemical to exert negative influence on offspring during the initial period of pregnancy, i.e., the period between conception and embryo formation. Teratogenicity means capability of a chemical to cause malformations and deviations in offspring postnatal development when a female body is exposed to this chemical during pregnancy [51].

Embryotoxic and teratogenic effects exerted by nanodisperse MnO_2 were examined and assessed at oral introduction with water in accordance with methodical guidelines on studying embryotoxic effects of chemicals at hygienic validation of their maximum permissible concentration in water of water objects [52]. The experiment was performed on white senior male and female Wistar rats with body weight equal to 200 ± 10 g (n = 90). All the animals before the experiment underwent 14-day quarantine and were placed in standard cages made of polypropylene, two animals in each. Rats were divided into three groups, 15 animals in each. Groups 1 and 2 were experimental ones, and group 3 was a control one. To get female rats pregnant, intact male rats and intact female rats were made to mate under control conditions during two estrous cycles. The day of sperm detection in vaginal smear of a female rat via microscopy was thought to be the first day of pregnancy. Nanodisperse MnO_2 water suspension was introduced into pregnant female rats daily one time a day via gastric tube from the first to the twenty-first pregnancy day in two doses: 2.50 mg/kg (1/1000 LD_{50}) and 0.25 mg/kg (1/10,000 LD_{50}). Control group of rats received distilled water. Changes in general condition and behavior of experimental animals were registered during the whole experiment. Rat's body weight was measured on the first, eighth, fourteenth and twenty-first day of pregnancy. Rats were taken out of the experiment via sparing euthanasia with carbon dioxide on the twenty-first day of pregnancy. Pregnant female rats were dissected just after euthanasia. Assessment was performed in two stages. On the first stage, overall disorders in fetus development (embryotoxicity) were assessed. On the second stage, the focus was on occurrence of congenital malformations in internal organs and skeletal system of fetuses (teratogenicity).

The experiment results showed that pregnant female rats from groups 1 and 2 had ordinary motion activity during the observation period. Innate reflexes and reactions to external irritants were normal and rats ate their forage willingly. Their fur was clean, shiny, and smooth. Visible mucous tunics were physiologically colored without any discharge. Appearance, behavior, and body weight dynamics of rats from experimental groups did not have any authentic discrepancies from the same parameters of rats from control group during the whole observation period. There were not any signs of animals intoxication or death in both experimental groups during the whole observation period. The examination results showed that all the embryotoxicity parameters (number of implantation points, number of viable fetuses, and number of resorptions) of pregnant female rats receiving nanodisperse MnO_2 water suspension via gastric tube formed during first to twenty-first day of pregnancy in doses equal to 2.5 and 0.25 mg/kg had no authentic discrepancies with the same parameters of rats from control group ($p > 0.05$). Fetuses from each litter did not have any visible external congenital malformations when being examined externally. There were not any authentic discrepancies between body weight or cranio-caudal body dimensions of fetuses from experimental and control groups.

There were no morphologic changes in internal organs or skeletal system of fetuses from groups 1 and 2 at intragastric introduction of nanodisperse MnO_2

water suspension into Wistar rats from first to twenty-first day of pregnancy; there were no discrepancies between morphologic characteristics of fetuses internal organs and fetuses skeletal system between experimental and control groups. Fetuses from experimental groups and control group had multilayer flat epidermis with increased number of layers up to eight cells; derma cells were spindle-shaped; fibers were tightly located and had numerous hair follicles. Subcutaneous fatty tissue was in the form of sporadic small lipocyte bunches (**Figure 17**). Small intestine wall is fully formed; limbic epithelium has characteristic appearance; Paneth cells are large and located not only in crypts bottom area, but also in villi epithelium. Beaker cells are sporadic (**Figure 18**).

Cartilaginous elements are mature; eosinophilic intracellular substance prevails in most cartilages (**Figures 19** and **20**).

There were numerous focuses of indirect and direct osteogenesis. Skeletal muscles are with small diameter of fibers and banding that is not clearly visible. Brain hemispheres cortex is cellular, layers are poorly differentiated and prevail over medulla. Cardiac histiocytes are with small section and large nucleuses. Fibers are spongy. Connective tissue content in cardiac muscle is minimal. Banding is not detected. Marrow is cellular; its bulk is represented by cells of erythropoetic type; there are no lipocytes.

Examining and assessing mutagenic activity of nanodisperse MnO_2 water suspension at oral introduction with water: micronucleus test is a widespread technique applied for assessing mutagenic activity of new unknown chemicals; the test was independently worked out and implemented by Heddle and Schmid in early 1970s [53]. Micronucleuses are small DNA-containing formations consisting of acentric chromosome fragments. During telophase, these fragments can become a part of daughter cells nucleuses or form singular or numerous micronucleuses in cytoplasm. The test is based on microscopic detection of cells with micronucleuses. Spontaneous frequency of cells with micronucleuses amounts to 0.1–0.2% [54].

Data on mutagenic activity, which nanosized MnO_2 particles, may be contradictory. The authors have not been able to find any research works proving apparent mutagenic properties of MnO_2 nanoparticles. At the same time, some experts state that MnO_2 nanoparticles are undoubtedly genotoxic "in vivo" [55]. There are data given by a number of researchers that manganese nanoparticles (52.1 ± 23.8 nm) at 24-hour exposure on PC-12 cells in concentration equal to 10 mg/cm^3 are able to inhibit PARK2 gene and tyrosine hydroxylase gene expression (The latter is an enzyme that catalyzes the first limiting stage of catecholamines synthesis, including dopamine.) It is detected that manganese nanoparticles enhance SNCA gene

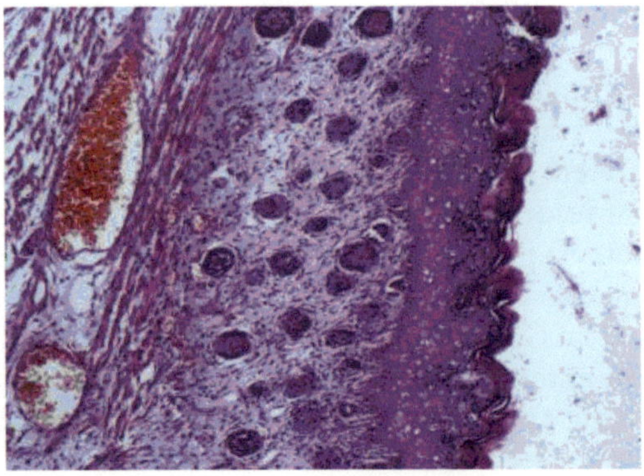

Figure 17.
Epidermis of Wistar rat fetus on the twenty-first day of pregnancy at intragastric introduction of nanodisperse MnO_2 water suspension via gastric tube. Painted with hematoxylin-eosin, magnification ×200 [10].

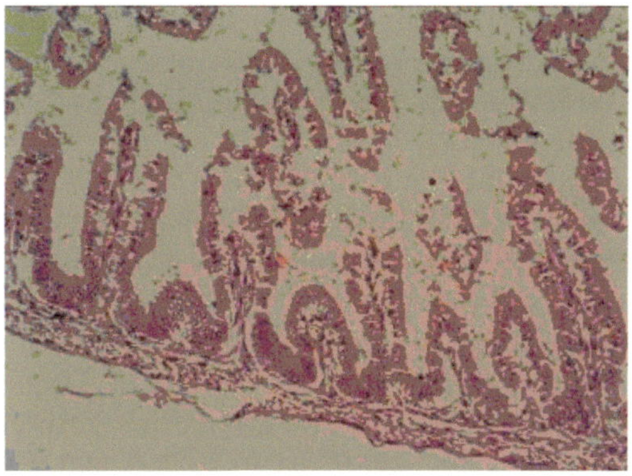

Figure 18.
Small intestine of a Wistar rat fetus on the twenty-first day of pregnancy at intragastric introduction of nanodisperse MnO_2 water suspension via gastric tube. Painted with hematoxylin-eosin, magnification ×200 [10].

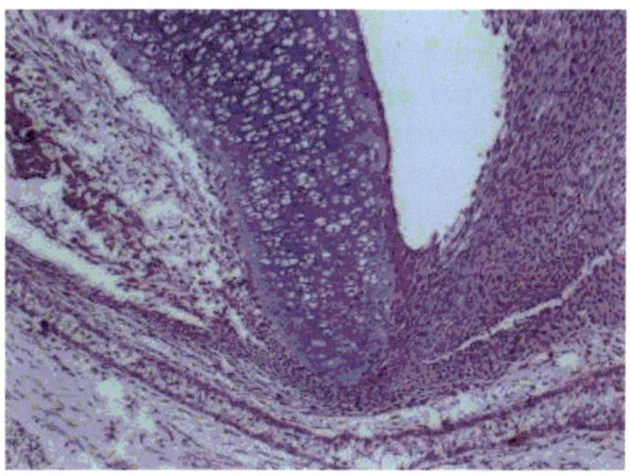

Figure 19.
Brainpan and brain of a Wistar rat fetus on the twenty-first day of pregnancy at intragastric introduction of nanodisperse MnO_2 water suspension via gastric tube. Painted with hematoxylin-eosin, magnification ×200 [10].

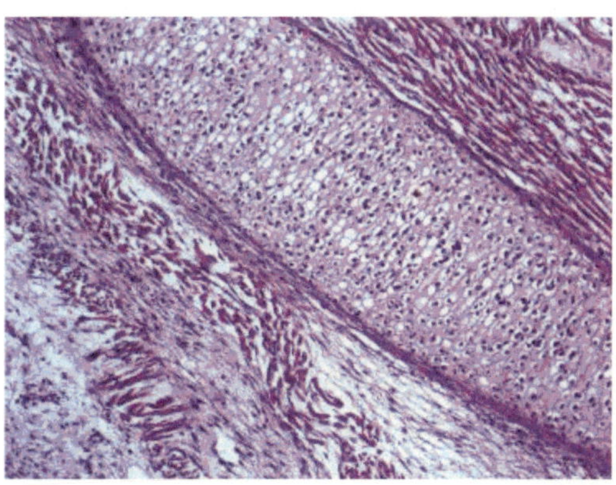

Figure 20.
Ribs and intercostal muscles of a Wistar rat fetus on the twenty-first day of pregnancy at intragastric introduction of nanodisperse MnO_2 water suspension via gastric tube. Painted with hematoxylin-eosin, magnification ×200 [10].

expression, which makes α-synucleins double in cells participating in various neurodegenerating disorders evolvement. After nanodisperse, MnO_2 was orally introduced into Wistar rats in doses equal to 300 and 1000 mg/kg during 28 days; there was an increased number of DNA damages in leucocytes, and also an increased number of micronucleuses and chromosome aberrations in marrow cells.

Potential mutagenic activity of nanodisperse MnO_2 water suspension in polychromatocytes (reticulocytes) of mammals marrow was assessed via micronucleus test [53]. The experiment was carried out on C57B1/6 white male mice with body weight equal to 20.0 ± 1.0 g (n = 24). The experiment lasted for 2 days. Experimental animals were divided into four groups (six animals in each); groups 1 and 2 were experimental ones, group 3 was negative control, and group 4 was positive control. Nanodisperse MnO_2 water suspension was once introduced via gastric tube in two doses: group 1 received 10.3 mg/kg (1/250 LD_{50}), group 2–5.15 mg/kg dose (1/500 LD_{50}), and group 3 (negative control)—distilled water in a volume equal to 0.2 cm^3 group 4 (positive control)—cyclophosphamide water suspension was once introduced intraperitoneally into mice from in a dose equal to 20 mg/kg in a volume equal to 0.2 cm^3. Cyclophosphamide is known to be cytogenetically active [13].

Thus, nanodisperse MnO_2 water suspension at a single intragastric introduction via gastric tube into C57B1/6 male mice in doses equal to 10.3 and 5.15 mg/kg does not cause increased micronucleuses formation in vivo and, consequently, does not have any mutagenic effects. As per other authors' data, there is no information on possible penetration of MnO_2 nanoparticles into cells nucleuses. It reduces the risk of direct contact between examined particles and cellular DNA [23]. DNA damage can occur through activation of lipid peroxidation and excessive AOF production from damaged membranes, which leads to cytokines induction (TNF-a tumor necrosis factor) and DNA damage. It can result in transcription factors activation, NF-KB in particular, which is responsible for polygenic expression. As a result, apoptotic mechanism is activated, or programmed cells death is inhibited, which can cause tumor activity [56, 57]. Some authors state that manganese nanoparticles (52.1 ± 23.8 nm) when exerting a 24-hour effect on PC-12 cells in concentration equal to 10 mg/cm^3 are able to inhibit PARK2 gene expression and gene of tyrosine hydroxylase (an enzyme that catalyzes the first limiting stage of catecholamine synthesis, dopamine included). It is proved that manganese nanoparticles enhance SNCA gene expression which leads to double increase in α-synucleins in cells taking part in evolvement of various neurodegenerating disorders. When nanodisperse MnO_2 was introduced into Wistar rats orally in doses equal to 300 and 1000 mg/kg during 28 days DNA damages in leucocytes increased, a number of micronucleuses and chromosome aberrations in marrow cells grew. These changes were accompanied with inhibition of various ATPases activity; here changes in ALAT, ASAT, and LDG activity in liver, kidneys, and blood serum were dose depending [44]. We could not find any research proving apparent mutagenic properties of MnO_2 particles. At the same time, a number of authors showed that MnO_2 nanoparticles had evident genotoxicity "in vivo" [43].

Examining and assessing gonadotoxic activity (screening) of MnO_2 oxide water suspension at oral introduction with water: gonadotoxicity of nanodisperse MnO_2 water suspension was examined on laboratory animals under subchronic experiment conditions in accordance with guidelines 2492-81 "On studying chemicals gonadotoxicity at hygienic standardization in water of water reservoirs" and international recommendations [58, 59]. The authors examined gonads of white male Wistar rats with body weight equal to 190 ± 20 g (n = 40). Experimental animals were divided into five groups, eight animals in each. Water suspension containing nanodisperse MnO_2 was introduced in a concentration equal to 36.0 ± 2.3 mg/cm^3, into animals from experimental groups via gastric tube once a day every day in following doses: group 1 received 257.7 mg/kg (1/10 LD_{50}), group 2–51.54 mg/kg (1/50 LD_{50}), group 3–10.3 mg/kg (1/250 LD_{50}), group 4–5.15 mg/kg (1/500 LD_{50}), and group 5 (control)—distilled water in a volume equal. The experiment lasted for 90 days. Animals euthanasia was accomplished with carbon dioxide. Then, a special instrument was applied to take out epididymis and make a longitudinal cut along it. Extraction of the epididymis in 10 cm^3 of 0.9% NaCl solution was performed during 2 minutes at room temperature being 22°C. Sperm quantity was calculated in Goryaev chamber. Specimens microscopy was performed with the use of MC 100X microscope (Micros, Austria). The task was to assess such functional and morphometric parameters as sperm mass, total sperm quantity, number of alive sperm, sperm mobility duration, osmotic and acidic resistance of sperm, relative quantity of sperm pathologies.

The obtained results revealed authentic 2.18 times decrease in sperm quantity in male rats from group 1 against the control group ($p < 0.05$). Male rats from group 2 had authentically 1.7 times lower quantity of sperm than rats from the control group. There were no authentic discrepancies in sperm number between male rats from groups 3, 4 and 5 and the control group. There was an authentic 1.2–1.3 times decrease in osmotic and acidic resistance of sperm in rats from groups 1 and 2 against the control group parameter ($p < 0.05$). There were no discrepancies in this parameter in rats from groups 3, 4 and 5 and the control group. Such morphological changes as sperm head, tail, and neck pathology occurred in groups 1 and 2 1.7–10.3 times more frequently than in the control group (**Figures 21** and **22**). This parameter in groups 3, 4, and 5 did not have any discrepancies with the control group parameter.

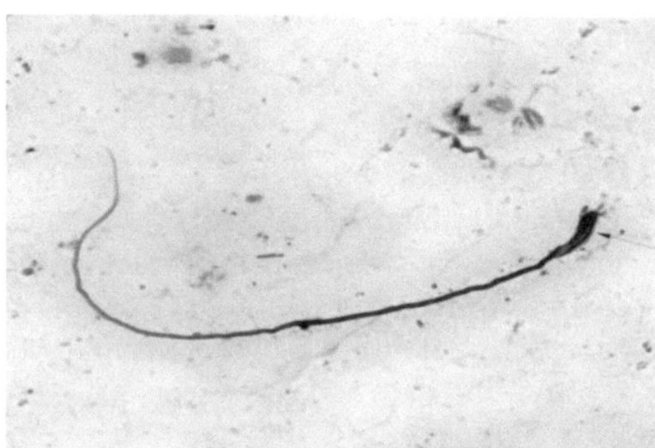

Figure 21.
A spermatozoon neck pathology in a male Wistar rat at oral introduction of nanodisperse MnO_2 in a dose equal to 51.54 mg/kg, magnification ×100 [55].

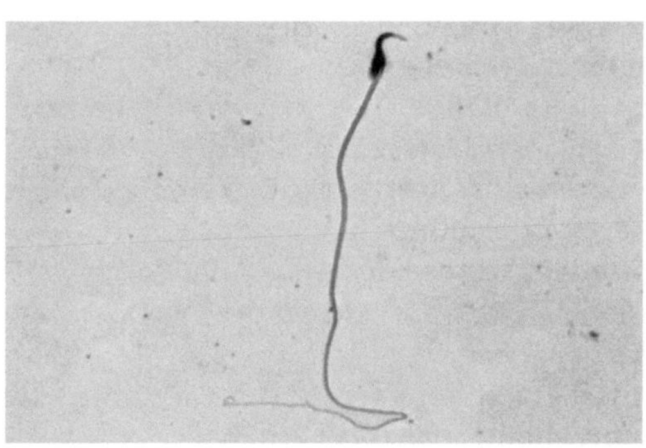

Figure 22.
A spermatozoon neck and head pathology in a male Wistar rat at oral introduction of nanodisperse MnO_2 in a dose equal to 257.7 mg/kg, magnification ×200 [55].

Therefore, nanodisperse MnO_2 water suspension does not exert any gonadotoxic effects on male Wistar rats when it is introduced into them via gastric tube during 90 days in doses equal to 10.3–5.15 mg/kg.

5. Conclusion

Contemporary research in nanotoxicology calls for studying and systemizing miscellaneous toxic effects exerted by new nanomaterials at various introduction ways and exposure period. Special attention is paid to determining target organs and negative effects caused by nanoparticles impacts, which do not occur after exposure to analog microparticles. To obtain comprehensive characteristics, one should study remote toxic effects such as embryotoxicity, gonadotoxicity, mutagenic activity occurrence, etc.

The authors conducted experimental research of nanodisperse MnO_2 water suspension at intragastric, inhalation, and skin-resorptive introduction into small rodents (mice and Wistar rats) with various exposure periods. It allowed to obtain a sufficiently profound and detailed characteristics of the toxic effects exerted by this substance, to determine the target organs and to reveal dose-dependent effects.

The obtained knowledge provides better understanding of toxic impact exerted by nanosized metal oxides, which have great potential of application in human activities. It is vital for working out efficient measures aimed at providing safety in production processes and in nanomaterials application.

Acknowledgements

The authors are grateful to specialists working at the multiphase disperse system laboratory of Technical Chemistry Institute (the Russian Academy of Sciences, Urals Branch), specialists working at Chemical Technologies Department of Perm National Research Polytechnic University, specialists working at Human Ecology and Life Activity Safety Department of Perm State National Research University, as they all contributed into providing data and materials for this edition.

Notation and abbreviations

IT	information technology
EU	European Union
SUN	sustainable nanotechnologies
GLP	good laboratory practice
XRD	X-ray diffraction
CAS	chemical abstracts service
IUPAC	International Union of Pure and Applied Chemistry
CTAB	cetyltrimethylammonium bromide
ILAR,	Institute for Laboratory Animal Research
DELS	division on earth and life studies
AOF	active oxygen forms
GSSG	oxidized glutathione form
GSH	reduced glutathione form
CL_{50}	concentration causing death of animals in quantity 50%
TCL_0	minimal toxic concentration
LDL_0	minimal lethal dose

LD_{50}	dose causing death of animals in quantity 50%
TL_{50}	time causing death of animals in quantity 50%
GABA	γ-aminobutyric acid
LP	lipid peroxidation
MDA	malonic dialdehyde
Cu/Zn-SOD	Cu/Zn-superoxide dismutase
OAS	overall antioxidant state
DNA	deoxyribonucleic acid

Author details

Nina Vladimirovna Zaitseva and Marina Alexandrovna Zemlyanova*
FBSI "Federal Scientific Center for Medical and Preventive Health Risk Management Technologies", Perm, Russian

*Address all correspondence to: zem@fcrisk.ru

IntechOpen

© 2019 The Author(s). Licensee IntechOpen. This chapter is distributed under the terms of the Creative Commons Attribution License (http://creativecommons.org/licenses/by/3.0), which permits unrestricted use, distribution, and reproduction in any medium, provided the original work is properly cited.

References

[1] Nanoindustry Analysis Results in CU and EES (Analytical Material) [Internet]. 2014. Available from: www.nanonewsnet.ru/news/2015/rezultaty-analiza-nanoindustrii-v-ramkakh-ts-eep [Accessed: 10 December 2018]

[2] Nanotechnologies Market in Russia [Internet]. 2017. Available from: http://prnews.ru/topic/analiz-rynka-nanotehnologij-v-rossii [Accessed: 11 December 2018]

[3] Onishchenko G. Security strategy in nanoindustry. Population Health and Environment. 2011;**5**:4-8

[4] Risk Assessment of Products of Nanotechnologies [Internet]. 2009. Available from: http://ec.europa.eu/health/ph_risk/committees/04_scenihr/docs/scenihr_o_023.pdf [Accessed: 11 December 2018]

[5] About Manganese [Internet]. 2017. Available from: https://www.americanelements.com/mn.html [Accessed: 11 December 2018]

[6] Portable Power Source [Internet]. 2009. Available from: http://bd.patent.su/2396000-2396999/pat/servl/servlet9ef1.html [Accessed: 11 December 2018]

[7] Dontsova EA, Budashov IA, Eremenko AV, Kurochkin IN. Hydrogen peroxide-sensitive amperometric sensor based on manganese dioxide nanoparticles. Nanotechnologies in Russia. 2008;**3**(7-8):510-520. DOI: 10.1134/s199507800807015x

[8] Detection of Nanomaterials which can be Potentially Dangerous for Human Health. MU 1.2.2522-09 [Internet]. 2009. Available from: www.gostrf.com/normadata/1/4293828/4293828130.pdf [Accessed: 11 December 2018]

[9] Sinha K, Suzuki K, Takahara M, Azuma H, Nonaka T, Fukumoto K. Mesostructured manganese oxide/gold nanoparticle composites for extensive air purification. Angewandte Chemie International. 2007;**46**:2891-2894. DOI: 10.1002/ange.200605048

[10] Zvezdin V, Zemlyanova M, Akafieva T. Inhalation toxicity of nanodispersed manganese oxide aerosol. Occupational Health and Industrial Ecology. 2015;**12**:13-16

[11] Guide for the Care and Use of Laboratory Animals. 8th ed. Washington: The National Academies Press; 2011. 220 p

[12] Manganese [Internet]. 2017. Available from: https://chem.libretexts.org/Textbook_Maps/Analytical_Chemistry/Supplemental_Modules_%28Analytical_Chemistry%29/Analytical_Chemiluminescence/2%3A_Chemiluminescence_Reagents/2.07%3A_Manganese [Accessed: 10 December 2018]

[13] Greg S, Singh K. Adsorption, Surface Area, Porosity. Moscow: Mir; 1984. 306 p

[14] Barrett E, Joyner L, Halenda P. The determination of pore volume and area distributions in porous substances. I. Computations from nitrogen isotherms. Journal of the American Chemical Society. 1951;**7**:373-380. DOI: 10.1021/ja01145a126

[15] Zaitseva N, Zemlianova M, Zvezdin V, Akafieva T, Saenko E. Acute inhalation toxicity of manganese oxide nanoparticles. Nanotechnologies in Russia. 2015;**10**(5-6):468-474. DOI: 10.1134/S1995078015030180

[16] Whitesides G, Eigler D, Anders R, et al. Nanotechnology in the next decade. In: Roco MC, Williams RS, Alivisatosa P, editors. Forecast Research. Moscow: Mir; 2002. 292 p

[17] Meynen V, Cool P, Vansant E. Verified syntheses of mesoporous materials. Microporous and Mesoporous Materials. 2009;**125**:170-223. DOI: 10.1016/j.micromeso.2009.03.046

[18] Gyrdasova O, Krasil'nikov V, Bazuev G. Synthesis of micro- and nanosized manganese oxides from hydrated manganese oxalates and products of their chemical modification with ethylene glycol. Russian Journal of Inorganic Chemistry. 2009;**7**:1035-1040. DOI: 10.1134/S0036023609070080

[19] Lison D, Lardot C, Huaux F, Zanetti G, Fubini B. Influence of partice surface area on the toxicity of insoluble manganese dioxide dusts. Archives of Toxicology. 1997;**71**(12):725-729. DOI: 10.1007/s002040050453

[20] Frick R, Müller-Edenborn B, Schlicker A, Rothen-Rutishauser B. Comparison of manganese oxide nanoparticles and manganese sulfate with regard to oxidative stress, uptake and apoptosis in alveolar epithelial cells. Toxicology Letters. 2011;**205**:163-172. DOI: 10.1016/j.toxlet.2011.05.1037

[21] Stefanescu D, Khoshnan A, Patterson P, Hering J. Neurotoxicity of manganese oxide nanomaterials. Journal of Nanoparticle Research. 2009;**11**(8):1957-1969. DOI: 10.1007/s11051-008-9554-1

[22] Elder A, Gelein R, Silva V, Feikert T, Opanashuk L, Carter J, et al. Translocation of inhaled ultrafine manganese oxide particles to the central nervous system. Environmental Health Perspectives. 2006;**114**:1172-1178. DOI: 10.1289/ehp.9030

[23] Ostiguy C, Asselin P, Malo S, Nadeau D. Prse en charge du manganisme d'origine professionnelle: Consensus d'un groupe d'experts: Rapport IRSST, No 416. Montreal: IRSST; 2005. 62 p

[24] Ostiguy C, Malo S, Asselin P. Synthese des connaissances scientifiques sur les risques d'atteinte a la sante suite a une exposition professionnelle au manganese: rapport IRSST, No 339. Montreal: IRSST; 2003. 41 p

[25] Afeseh Ngwa H, Kanthasamy A, Gu Y, Fang N. Manganese nanoparticle activates mitochondrial dependent apoptotic signaling and autophagy in dopaminergic neuronal cells. Toxicology and Applied Pharmacology. 2011;**256**:227-240. DOI: 10.1016/j.taap.2011.07.018

[26] Horváth E, Máté Z, Takács S, Pusztai P, Sápi A, Kónya Z, et al. General and electrophysiological toxic effects of manganese in rats following subacute Administration in Dissolved and Nanoparticle Form. The Scientific World Journal. 2012:1-7. DOI: 10.1100/2012(6)/520632

[27] Crittenden P, Filipov N. Manganese-induced potentiation of in vitro pro-inflammatory cytokine production by activated microglial cells is associated with persistent activation of p38 MAPK. Toxicology in Vitro. 2008;**22**: 18-27. DOI: 10.1016/j.tiv.2007.07.004

[28] Sárközi L, Horváth E, Kónya Z, Kiricsi I. Subacute intratracheal exposure of rats to manganese nanoparticles: Behavioral, electrophysiological, and general toxicological effects. Inhalation Toxicology. 2009;**1**:83-91. DOI: 10.1080/08958370902939406

[29] Wang J, Rahman M, Duhart H, Newport G. Expression changes of dopaminergic system-related genes in PC12 cells induced by manganese, silver, or copper nanoparticles. Neurotoxicology. 2009;**30**:926-933. DOI: 10.1016/j.neuro.2009.09.005

[30] Oberdorster G, Sharp Z, Atudorei V. Translocation of inhaled ultrafine particles to the brain. Inhalation

Toxicology. 2004;**16**:437-445. DOI: 10.1080/08958370490439597

[31] Nanotechnology KJ. Piecing together the puzzle of risk. Controversies in Science and Technology. 2011;**3**:243-255. DOI: 10.1089/9781934854204.243

[32] Laohaudomchok W, Lin X, Herrick RF, Fang SC, Cavallari JM, Shrairman R, et al. Neuropsychological effects of low-level manganese exposure in welders. Neurotoxicology. 2011;**32**(2):171-179. DOI: 10.1016/j.neuro.2010.12.014

[33] Li T, Shi T, Li X, Zeng S, Yin L, Pu Y. Effects of nano-MnO_2 on dopaminergic neurons and the spatial learning capability of rats. International Journal of Environmental Research and Public Health. 2014;**11**(8):7918-7930. DOI: 10.3390/ijerph110807918

[34] Zemlyanova M, Zvezdin V, Akafieva T. Inhalation toxicity of nanodispersed manganese oxide aerosol. Labor Medicine and Industrial Ecology. 2015;**12**:13-17

[35] Amatucci GG, Pereira N. Fluoride based electrode materials for advanced energy storage devices. Journal of Fluorine Chemistry. 2007;**128**:243-262. DOI: 10.1016/j.jfluchem.2006.11.016

[36] Hua M, Zhang S, Pan B, Zhang W, Lv L, Zhang Q. Heavy metal removal from water/wastewater by nanosized metal oxides: A review. Journal of Hazardous Materials. 2012;**211-212**:317-331. DOI: 10.1016/j.jhazmat.2011.10.016

[37] Zaitseva N, Zemlyanova M, Zvezdin V, Akafyeva T. Biological effects of manganese oxide nanoparticles after peroral intake. Journal of Pharmacy and Nutrition Sciences. 2013;**3**(4):231-237

[38] Zaitseva N, Zemlyanova M, Zvezdin V, Saenko E, Tarantin A, Makhmudov R, et al. Toxicological-hygienic assessment of nanodisperse and microdisperse manganese oxide safety (III, IV). Nutrition Issues. 2012;**81**(5):13-19

[39] Shtabskiy B. Quantitative assessment of cumulation. Hygiene and Sanitary. 1973;**8**:24-28

[40] Mousavi Z, Hassanpourezatti M, Najafizadeh P, Rezagholian S, Safi Rhamanifar M, Nosrati N. Effects of subcutaneous injection MnO_2 micro- and nanoparticles on blood glucose level and lipid profile in rat. The Iranian Journal of Medical Sciences. 2016;**41**(6):518-524

[41] Zaitseva N, Zemlyanova M, Zvezdin V, Akafyeva T, Mazunina D, Dovbyish A. Effects of subchronic exposure manganese oxide nanoparticles on the central nervous system, lipid peroxidation and antioxidant enzymes in rats. Health Risk Analysis. 2014;**4**:66-77

[42] Sakon S, Xue X, Takekawa M, Sasazuki T, Okazaki T, Kojima Y, et al. NF-kB inhibits TNF-induced accumulation of ROS that mediate prolonged MAPK activation and necrotic cell death. The EMBO Journal. 2003;**22**(15):3898-3909. DOI: 10.1093/emboj/cdg379

[43] Tin-Tin W-S, Fujimaki H. Nanoparticles and neurotoxicity. Journal of Molecular Science. 2011;**12**:6267-6280. DOI: 10.3390/ijms12096267

[44] Singh SP, Kumari M, Kumari SI, Rahman MF. Toxicity assessment of manganese oxide micro and nanoparticles in Wistar rats after 28 days of repeated oral exposure. Journal of Applied Toxicology. 2013;**33**(10):1165-1179. DOI: 10.1002/jat.2887

[45] Mousavi Z, Hassanpourezatti M, Najafizadeh P, Rezagholian S, Rhamanifar NN. Effects of subcutaneous injection MnO_2 micro- and nanoparticles on blood glucose level and lipid profile in rat. Iranian Journal of Medical Sciences. 2016;**41**(6):518-524

[46] Ghaedi S, Hassanpour-Ezatti M, Naji T, Rahmanifar MS. Comparison of tissue damages resulting from chronic administration of manganese dioxide nano-and microparticles on the liver, kidneys and testes of rats. Modares Journal of Medical Sciences: Pathobiology. 2014;**16**(4):67-81

[47] Deng Q, Liu J, Li Q, Ket C, Liu Z, Shen Y, et al. Interaction of occupational manganese exposure and alcohol drinking aggravates the increase of liver enzyme concentrations from a cross-sectional study in China. Environmental Health. 2013;**12**:30. DOI: 10.1186/1476-069X-12-30

[48] Onishhenko GG, Tutel'jan VA, Hotimchenko SA, Gmoshinskij IV, et al. Toxicologic-Hygienic Assessment of Nanomaterial Safety: MU 1.2.2520-09. Moscow: Federal Center for Hygiene and Epidemiology of Rospotrebnadzor; 2009. 43 p

[49] Onishhenko GG, Bragina IV, Aksenova OI, Zavistjaeva TJu, Assessment et al. Order when Assessing Toxic Effects Exerted by Nanomaterials on Laboratory Animals. MU1.2.2869-11. Moscow: Federal center for Hygiene and Epidemiology of Rospotrebnadzor; 2011. 23 p

[50] Zaitseva N, Zemlyanova M, Zvezdin V, Sayenko Y. Toxicological and hygienic safety assessment of the aqueous suspension of nano-dispersed silicon dioxide, synthesized using liquid-crystal templating. Health Risk Analysis. 2013;**1**:65-72

[51] Sanockij I, Sidorov K, editors. Russian Glossary of Selected Terms from Preventive Toxicology. Moscow: Centr mezhdunar. proektov GKNT; 1982. 68 p

[52] Methodical Guidelines on Studying Embryotoxic Effects of Chemicals at Hygienic Validation of their Maximum Permissible Concentration in Water of Water Objects. MU 2926-83. [Internet]. 1983. Available from: http://www.normacs.ru/Doclist/doc/11NEJ.html [Accessed: 11 December 2018]

[53] Ledebur MV, Schmid W. The micronucleus test methodological aspects. Mutation Research/Fundamental and Molecular Mechanisms of Mutagenesis. 1973;**19**(1):109-117. DOI: 10.1016/0027-5107(73)90118-8

[54] Manual on experimental (preclinical) study of new pharmacological substances. Edited by a corresponding member of the RAMS, Prof. R.N. Habriev. Moscow: Methodical Guidelines; 2005. 832 p. Available from: https://elibrary.ru/item.asp?id=19116235&

[55] Minigalieva IA, Katsnelson BA, Privalova LI, Sutunkova MP, Gurvich VB, Shur VY, et al. Attenuation of combined nickel (II) oxide and manganese (II, III) oxide nanoparticles' adverse effects with a complex of bioprotectors. International Journal of Molecular Sciences. 2015;**16**(9):22555-22583. DOI: 10.3390/ijms160922555

[56] Pahl H. Activators and target genes of Rel/NF–kB transcription factors. Oncogene. 1999;**18**:6853-6866. DOI: 10.1038/sj.onc.1203239

[57] Takizawa H, Ohtoshi T, Kawasaki S, Kohyama T, Desaki M, Kasama T, et al. Diesel exhaust particles induce NF-kB activation in human bronchial epithelial cells in vitro: Importance in cytokine transcription. Journal of Immunology. 1999;**162**:4705-4711. DOI: 0022-1767/99/$02.00

[58] Guidelines for the Study Gonadotoxic Action of Chemical Substances in Hygienic Rationing

of Water Reservoirs. MU 2492-81 [Internet]. 1981. Available from: http://docs.cntd.ru/document/675400365 [Accessed: 11 December 2018]

[59] ICH Harmonised Tripartite Guideline [Internet]. 1993. Available from: https://www.ich.org/fileadmin/Public_Web_Site/ICH_Products/Guidelines/Efficacy/E7/Step4/E7_Guideline.pdf [Accessed: 11 December 2018]

Chapter 7

Intracellular Iron Concentration and Distribution Have Multiple Effects on Cell Cycle Events

Paul Seligman and Gamini Siriwardana

Abstract

Iron is essential for numerous cellular reactions that require oxygen transfer. Iron deficiency is a common problem in humans and is the most common nutritional disease worldwide. However, excess cellular iron can be toxic. Maintenance of iron hemostasis utilizes specialized pathways responsible for iron transport, iron uptake by cells, and appropriate cellular distribution of iron for utilization or storage. This chapter reviews how iron depletion is associated with inhibition of cellular proliferation and cell cycle arrest at different parts of the cell cycle. These effects are based on the effective chelation of iron, and more importantly on differences in various tissue responses to both iron depletion and iron toxicity. These differences may explain why in some tissues, particularly rapidly growing cancer cells, iron depletion causes cell cycle arrest and apoptosis, a form of programed cell death. Other neoplastic tissues are more prone to the toxic effects of iron, which can induce autophagic cell death (termed ferroptosis) via reactive oxygen species resulting in lysosomal degradation of cellular constituents. An appreciation of these differences can be utilized by novel pharmaceutical agents discussed below designed to treat specific cancers.

Keywords: cell cycle, iron chelation, redox, ROS, ferroptosis

1. Introduction

Iron is mainly used in oxygen transfer reactions necessary for moving oxygen to tissues by heme moieties including hemoglobin and myoglobin, enzymes necessary for oxidative phosphorylation, and oxygen transfer reactions by enzymes containing iron sulfur compounds [1, 2]. Compared to other essential micronutrients, iron is found in relatively high (micromolar) concentrations in tissues and serum. Although essential for these oxygen transfer reactions, excess iron is toxic [1–4]. Therefore complex pathways have evolved to maintain proper iron hemostasis utilizing specialized proteins responsible for iron transport, iron uptake by cells, and appropriate cellular distribution of iron for utilization or storage [1, 2]. Based on iron needs, promoters control transcription of proteins involved in iron homeostasis. Additionally, specialized elements regulate mRNA translation called iron regulatory elements act in a coordinated manner to rapidly regulate concentrations of transferrin receptor (necessary for transferrin bound iron cellular uptake) when more iron is needed, and ferritin, (the iron storage protein) when the cellular iron

IntechOpen

concentration is high [1, 4]. Ferritin concentrations both intracellular, and small amounts of secreted ferritin found in serum, are increased when there is excess iron, as well as in inflammatory conditions such as infections or cancer, presumably to inhibit iron utilization as well as protect against cellular iron toxicity. Transferrin receptor density is much higher in cells that require more iron, such as cells that synthesize hemoglobin and cells that are actively proliferating [5].

Agents that interfere with iron uptake or iron utilization have been used to treat cancer. One such agent used in limited clinical studies is gallium, a relatively inert metal that binds to transferrin and inhibits cellular iron uptake and utilization [6]. Another is the iron chelator deferioxamine (DFO) used in the treatment of neuroblastoma [7]. DFO has been considered the "gold standard" as a treatment for iron overload [1, 4]. However, newer iron chelators are not only more practical (oral gastrointestinal absorption) but have improved iron chelation efficacy and a more rapid onset of action. They are also lipophilic, however, and hence can potentially confound other biologic processes [8], including lipid peroxidation and autophagy if used for iron depletion only. Lipophilicity may have more potential for cancer treatment, particularly in combination with carefully chosen chemotherapeutic agents [8, 9], since utilizing the iron chelation effect alone combined with agents that specifically inhibit DNA synthesis, for example, may result in less combined efficacy [10].

Iron, therefore, is a requirement for cellular proliferation, particularly rapidly growing cells (including cancer cells). Clinical measurements of iron status in epidemiologic studies have shown a lower incidence of cancer in iron depleted individuals [11, 12], better survival in patients whose tumors retain less iron, and a higher incidence in those with or at risk for iron overload [13, 14].

Cellular iron depletion caused by the use of iron chelators *in vitro* is associated with inhibition of cellular proliferation attributable to cell cycle arrest [15–17]. Initially the deficit was ascribed only to inhibition of ribonucleotide reductase (RNR) an iron dependent enzyme necessary for DNA synthesis. The iron facilitates formation of a tyrosyl free radical at the active site of the M2 protein subunit of RNR [18, 19]. Hydroxyurea (HU), a cancer chemotherapy agent well absorbed after oral administration, is converted to a free radical nitroxide *in vivo* and quenches the tyrosyl free radical of RNR. Inhibition of RNR is associated with an early S phase block (sometimes described as a G1/S block). Some studies have indicated that the S phase block associated with ribonucleotide reductase inhibition might be distinguished from a G1 block, which may also occur with iron depletion [20, 21].

2. Iron depletion causes inhibition of cellular proliferation and at least two blocks in the cell cycle

More recently, an important advantage for studying cell cycle events has been the development of newer reagents that better pinpoints these events. In particular, antibodies that recognize cell cycle specific phosphorylation events, such as kinase activation status, have proven quite useful. Our more recent studies have shown that the two blocks caused by HU vs. iron chelation can be distinguished by different cell cycle events. In these studies we utilized neuroblastoma cell lines that are relatively sensitive to growth inhibition by iron depletion [22]. Although several other cell lines have shown both G1 and S phase inhibition by iron chelation, we chose the SKNSH neuroblastoma line because of reproducible predictable growth rates as well as consistently diploid chromosomal makeup and consistent contact inhibition with greater than 90% of cells in (G0) G1. SKNSH cells uniformly respond to various stimuli including those that promote cell proliferation. Examples of these promoters include simply subculture into serum containing media. These conditions make the cell line particularly useful for the study of very early cell cycle events after the stimulus for proliferation.

In these studies, timed experiments used sequential blocking by specific agents including aphidicolin (aph) (DNA polymerase inhibitor causing G1/S block), HU (RNR inhibition), specific kinase inhibitors (i.e., psrc or pcdk2 inhibition), and DFO. Cells were > 90 in G1 phase due to contact inhibition and stimulated to proliferate by subculture in "fresh" medium in 10% fetal calf serum (FCS) Timed studies were performed at the time of the proliferation stimulus, the addition of these specific agents, and "release" (wash out) of these agents. "Release medium" containing heat inactivated FCS was added after the attached cells were extensively washed with phosphate buffered saline. In previous studies we found that medium such as RPMI (supposedly with no added iron salts or FCS) actually contains 1–2 μmol/L of contaminating iron salts and about 0.6 μmol iron/L presumably bound to the transferrin in fetal calf serum. The initial DFO effect was associated with G1 arrest, persistence of cyclin E protein but inhibition of cyclin E/cdk2 complex activity, and no measurable cyclin A protein. DFO washout and media replacement resulted in the rapid disappearance of cyclin E (**Figure 1**). The block by aph was associated with a slight widening of G1 phase suggesting arrest at G1/S, but more importantly cyclin A protein was evident with no discernible cyclin E present. In contrast HU treatment exhibited a block in early to mid-S phase. DFO added slightly before release from aph showed cell cycle changes similar to HU suggesting that this block was due to RNR inhibition (**Figure 2**). These results were confirmed by studies of a unique cell line with a much higher rate of proliferation that consistently was resistant to the G1 effects of iron depletion. It also exhibited persistent cyclin A protein, perhaps due to less contact inhibition.

Recent studies have indicated at least one reason for the G1 block is an iron requirement for psrc activation. Src is inactive in the absence of iron as demonstrated by both lack of phosphorylation of Y416 (active site) and persistent phosphorylation at the inactivating Y527. Progression of mammalian cells into S phase from late G1 also requires the activation of cdk2 by cyclin E. Cdk2 bound to P27 is in an inactive state. In our studies, although the rapid activation of src with iron repletion was short-lived, it was rapidly followed by P27 degradation allowing

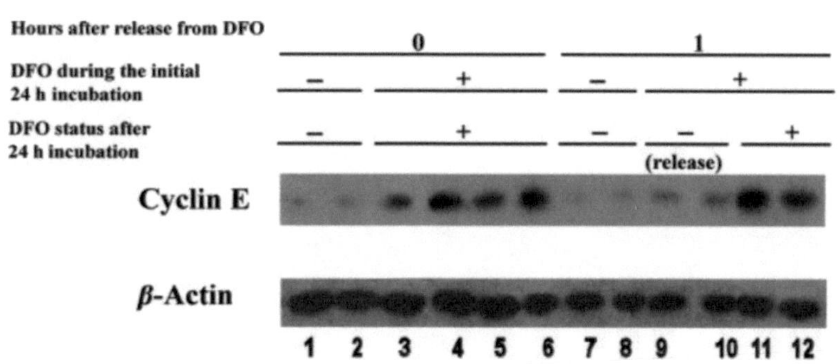

Figure 1.
This figure and legend were taken from Siriwardana and Seligman [23]. Cyclin E levels decrease after 1 h of release from the DFO block. Confluent neuroblastoma cells were serum starved for 24 h then split and plated into media, one set with DFO (lanes 3–6, 9–12) and one with no DFO (lanes 1–2, 7–8) and were incubated for 24 h. After 24 h, one set of cells that was in DFO was replaced with CM (release). Medium in the others were replaced with CM (continuously in medium without DFO). The medium in all plates was aspirated 1 h later and the cells were lysed using 200 μL of hot SDS loading buffer. Forty microliter samples of the lysate were separated by 10% SDS-PAGE and the proteins were transferred to PVDF membranes. This was first probed for cyclin E. Then the membrane was stripped and was probed for β-actin. All treatments were conducted in duplicate.

for activation of cdk2 by its phosphorylation at THR 160 presumably resulting in activation of the cdk2/cyclin E complex (**Figures 3–5**).

These events in turn were followed by rapid disappearance of cyclin E protein, presumably due to cdk2/cyclin E complex activity, and appearance of cyclin A protein allowing cells to proceed into and through S phase. Inhibition of src kinase activity may account for decreased downstream events ascribed to iron depletion in other cell lines including inhibition of cyclin D synthesis [25], an event not seen in SKNSH due to constitutive expression of cyclin D [23]. For example, we have found that the S phase kinase associated protein (Skp2), which is responsible for promoting p27 degradation, was not upregulated in the presence of DFO [26]. In contrast, p27 was not degraded after release from the iron block in the presence of the proteasome inhibitor MG132 (unpublished data). Other studies have asserted lack of p27 degradation does not allow for activation of cdk2, but more recently iron chelation was found to cause specific inactivation of cdk2 by persistence of the p21 inhibitor [27].

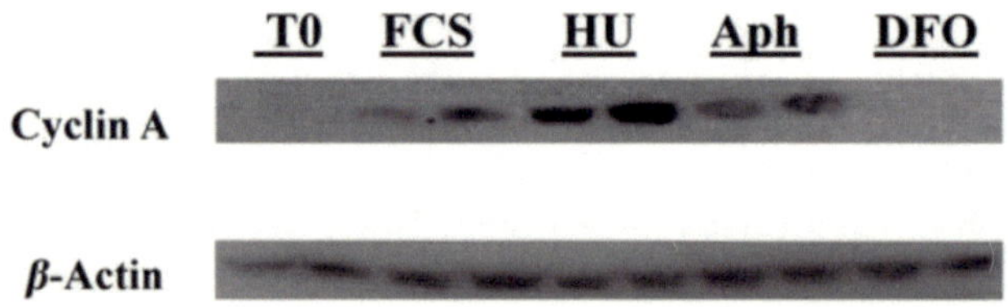

Figure 2.
This figure and legend was adapted from Siriwardana and Seligman [23]. Cyclin A is absent in DFO-treated neuroblastoma cells but occurs in cells arrested with aphidicolin or hydroxyurea. Serum starved neuroblastoma cells for 24 h were subcultured in CM (FCS), or RPMI/10% FCS with hydroxyurea, aphidicolin or DFO. The dishes were incubated for 24 h and the cells were harvested in 0.5 mL of cold PBS, a 50 μL portion of cells was used for FACS and the rest were centrifuged, supernatant removed and added with 200 μL of hot SDS loading buffer. Forty microliter samples of the lysate were separated by 10% SDS-PAGE and the proteins were transferred to PVDF membranes. This was probed for cyclin A. Then, the membrane was stripped and was probed for β-actin. All treatments were conducted in duplicate.

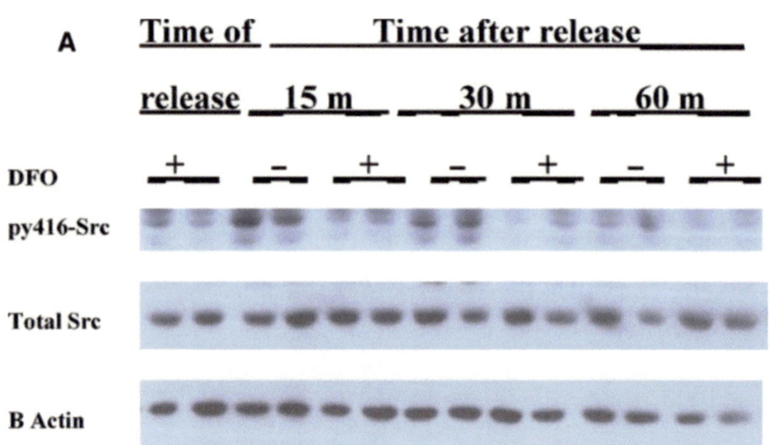

Figure 3.
This figure and legend were adapted from Siriwardana and Seligman [24].Confluent SKNSH cells were sub-cultured into RPMI/10% heat-inactivated FCS with 100 μm DFO and incubated. After 20 h the medium was replaced with new medium containing no DFO and 10% heat deactivated FCS. The cells were harvested at regular intervals beginning 15 min after aspirating the medium and adding hot SDS loading buffer. Westerns were performed as described and Src p416 levels were determined. Thereafter, the blot was stripped and probed for B Actin. Each treatment was conducted in duplicate. Based on densitometry, pSrc/B-Actin (average of duplicates) for RM vs. RM with DFO, respectively. 0 time 0.35 vs. 0.29; 15 min 0.78 vs. 0.28; 30 min 0.55 vs. 0.21; 60 min 0.31 vs. 0.26.

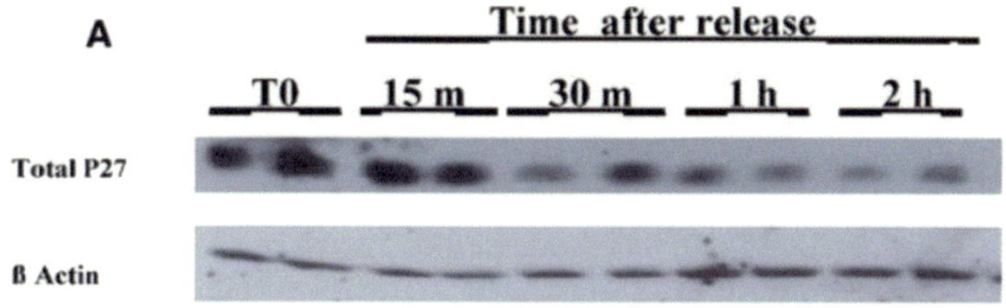

Figure 4.
This figure and legend were adapted from Siriwardana and Seligman [24]. Total p27 levels decrease rapidly after release from the DFO block. Confluent SKNSH cells were sub-cultured into RPMI/10% FCS with 100 µm DFO and incubated. After 20 h the medium was replaced with new medium as RM. The cells were harvested at regular intervals beginning 15 min after aspirating the medium and adding hot SDS loading buffer. Westerns were performed as described and (total) p27 levels were determined. Thereafter, the blot was stripped and probed for B Actin. Each treatment was conducted in duplicate.

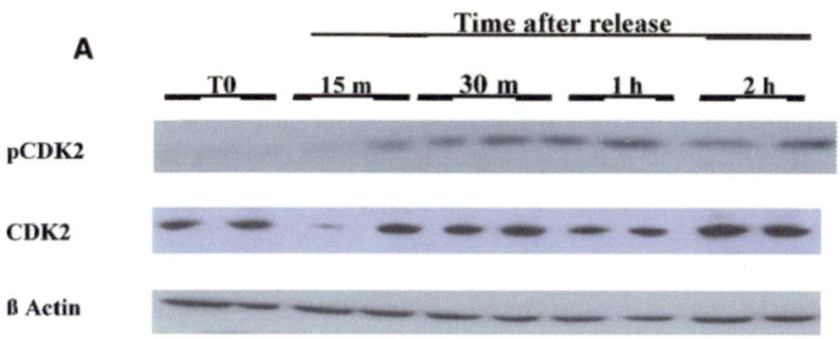

Figure 5.
This figure and figure legend were adapted from Siriwardana and Seligman [24]. Confluent SKNSH cells were sub-cultured into RPMI/10% FCS (CM) with 100 um DFO and incubated. After 20 h the medium was replaced with new medium containing no DFO and 10% heat deactivated FCS (RM). The cells were harvested at regular intervals beginning at 15 min after RM added, the medium was aspirated and hot SDS loading buffer was added. Westerns were performed as described and pcdk2 levels were determined. Thereafter, the blot was stripped and probed for total cdk2 and then B Actin. Each treatment was conducted in duplicate.

In recent unpublished studies we have found evidence that cells blocked at G1/S by aphidicolin, a DNA polymerase inhibitor, do not proceed into S phase if the cells are depleted of iron. The cells remain in G1/S, a block distinguished from both the block in G1 associated with iron depletion alone, as well as the block associated with RNR inhibition by iron depletion. Progression of cells into S phase after release from aphidicolin is prevented with the use of DFO and not with the src inhibitor, AZD, suggesting iron depletion has an additional cell cycle arrest mechanism independent of src inhibition by iron depletion causing G1 arrest as well as the later arrest due to inhibition of RNR caused by iron depletion (similar to the HU arrest),

Cells were incubated in aph or HU in RPMI with 10% F CS for 24 h. Then the cells received either no addition, DFO, or AZD for 16 h ahead of release from aph or HU. This 16 h time point was chosen because our previous studies have shown that DFO required at least several hours to effectively remove the "chelatable" cellular iron, a reference to iron that is readily bioavailable, as opposed to, for example, iron stored in ferritin. At 16 h (a total of about 40 h) these time periods were chosen because of extensive studies detailing the rate of proliferation of SKNSH cells with or without added agents, to ensure <10% of the cells are dead (by trypan blue exclusion), and allow time for the vast majority of cells to exhibit the block desired, including allowing a minority of the cells to "recycle" after division to the area of the block. The cells were released from aph or HU to medium, RPMI (10%FCS) with no addition, with DFO or with AZD. The cells were harvested 6 h later and a florescent activated cell sorter was used in order to measure DNA content utilizing propidium iodide.

Figures 6–10 shows DNA profiles of cells treated as indicated above. Our previous studies documented that effective chelation of intracellular iron by DFO *in vitro* took at least several hours [20]. Therefore cells incubated in aph for 2 days exhibited the expected G1/S block and after adding "release" medium with no addition for 6 h cells were almost exclusively in early and mid-S phase (**Figures 6** and 7). Aph treatment with DFO added only one half hour before "wash out" [so then is the DFO also washed out?], even with the DFO added to the release medium for 6 h, showed an almost identical profile as cells without DFO added (**Figure 8**). However, when DFO was added 16 h before release, and the cells were released in medium containing DFO for 6 h the profile showed cells still arrested in G1/S (**Figures 9** and **10**).

This effect of iron chelation by DFO causing a block at G1/S is distinct from inhibition of src kinase by DFO treatment in G1 phase. Treatment with the specific src kinase inhibitor AZD 0530 (AZD) showed almost identical DNA profile results as DFO treatment during G1 phase [24]. When AZD was added to cells 16 h before release from Aph and continued in release medium (no addition), 6 h later the profile showed results similar to no AZD treatment with the vast majority of cells in S phase (**Figures 11** and **12**).

Cells in HU for 48 h at the time of release into fresh medium are in early S phase, indicating inhibition of DNA synthesis caused by depletion of deoxyribonucleotides due to inhibition of RNR. These cells will proceed through S phase 6 h later after wash out (**Figures 13** and **14**). However, when DFO is added to the HU containing media 16 h before release most of the cells appear to be in G1/S phase, at the time of release. Moreover, when the same cells are released into medium containing DFO, the vast majority have still have not entered S phase 6 h later, although there are still a few cells in early S.

Studies using inhibitors of cdk2 activity were performed to determine its requirement for cell cycle progression. We hypothesized that iron depletion caused by DFO at G1 and S phase was not an effect of RNR inhibition, but a different process necessary to exit G1/S phase. We therefore assessed the effects of two cdk2 inhibitors JNJ7706621 (JNJ) and BMS 387032 (BMS). Both inhibitors affect the activity of other cyclin dependent kinases but have some specificity for cdk2. These agents have been used in humans as investigational study drugs in cancer protocols (supported by Johnson and Johnson and Bristol Myers Squibb respectively).

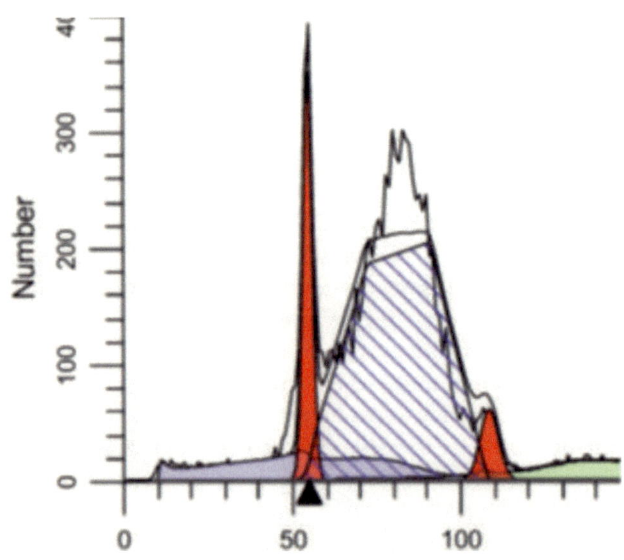

Figure 6.
Aph at time of release.

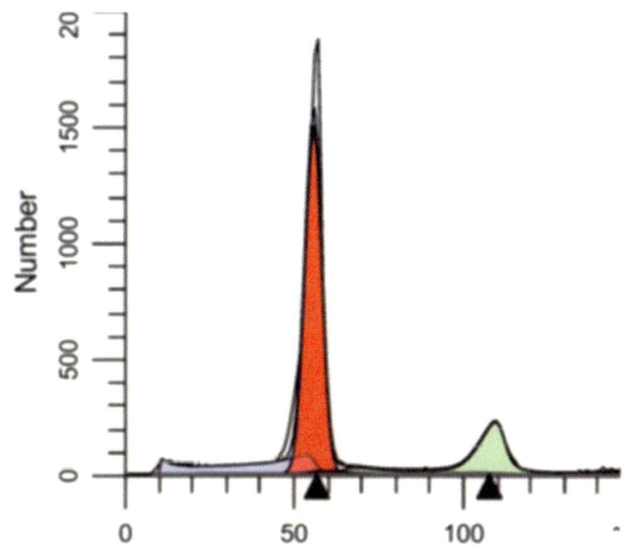

Figure 7.
Six hours after release into medium (no addition).

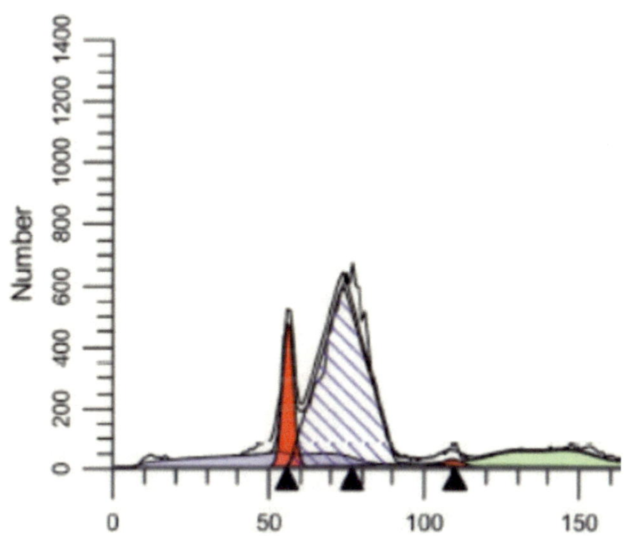

Figure 8.
Aph 6 h after release with DFO in release medium but no DFO added before.

As expected adding both inhibitors to cells treated with aph overnight, and maintaining their presence upon aph release (6 h) showed persistent G1/S phase arrest (**Figures 15** and **16**). Moreover, when BMS [28] was added to HU treated cells overnight and maintained after release, about 85% of cells remained in G1/S. The percentage of cells in S and G2/M phase when JNJ was added under these conditions showed about 20–25% of cells in S and G2/M phase, perhaps showing a different effect of BMS under these conditions (data not shown).

In conclusion the studies shown in **Figures 6–16** indicate there is a third cell cycle block caused by iron depletion distinct from the G1 block associated with psrc inhibition and the early to mid—S phase block caused by inhibition of RNR. The third putative block similar to the G1/S block seen with DNA polymerase inhibition (Aph) and with the less specific cdk2 inhibitors (**Figure 17**).

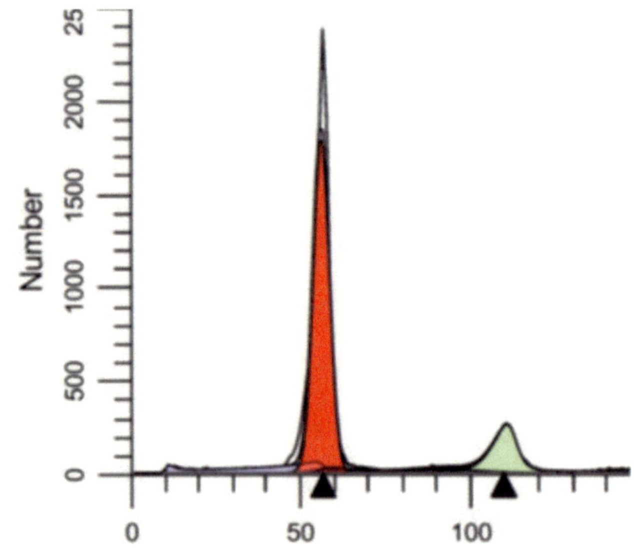

Figure 9.
Aph at time of release with DFO added for 16 h before rebase.

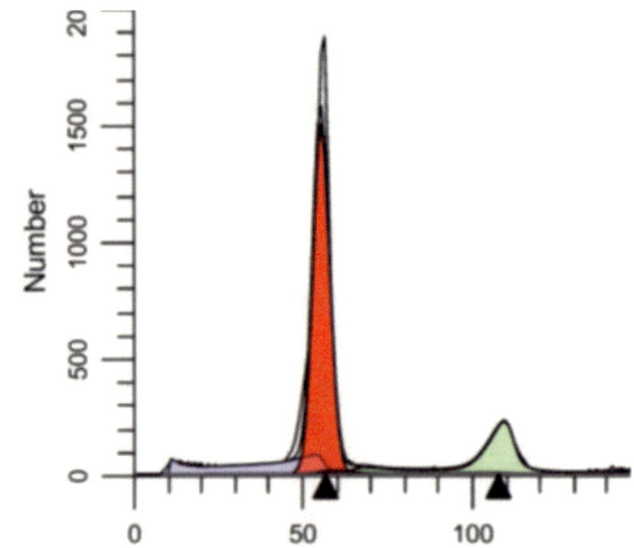

Figure 10.
Six hours after release from aph and DFO with DFO in release medium. [G1-88%, S-5%, G2/M-5% "dead" cells in this case are shown mostly to the left of the G1 peak and are discounted].

In initial Western blot experiments we found that DFO reduces the active cdk2 and cyclin A, whereas src inhibition does not. Cells were incubated in aph for 24 h, followed by addition of DFO for 16 h. Cells treated with aph had measurable src kinase, cdk2 kinase and cyclin A protein as shown in our prior studies. As expected, cells treated with AZD showed decreased src kinase activity in both incubation times but adequate levels of cyclin A and cdk2 kinase. Taken together these results strongly suggest that another block caused by iron depletion is associated with an event that occurs after src kinase activity, but before the initiation of DNA synthesis.

However, further studies need to be performed to assess the significance and longer-term effects of the decreased cyclin A and pcdk2 with the longer DFO

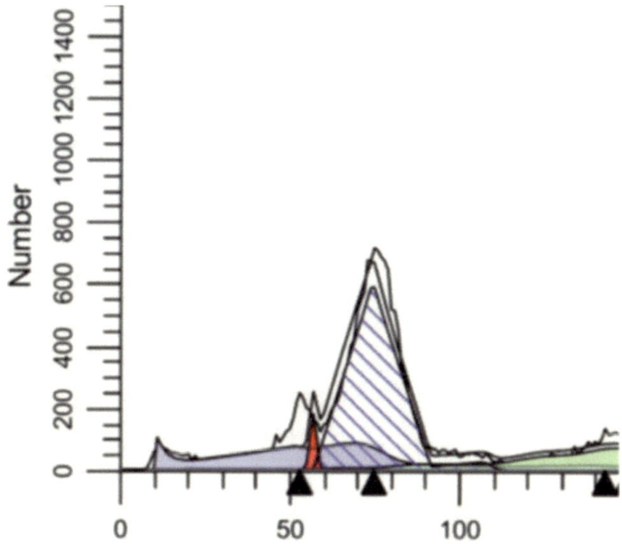

Figure 11.
Aph time of release with AZD added 16 h before release.

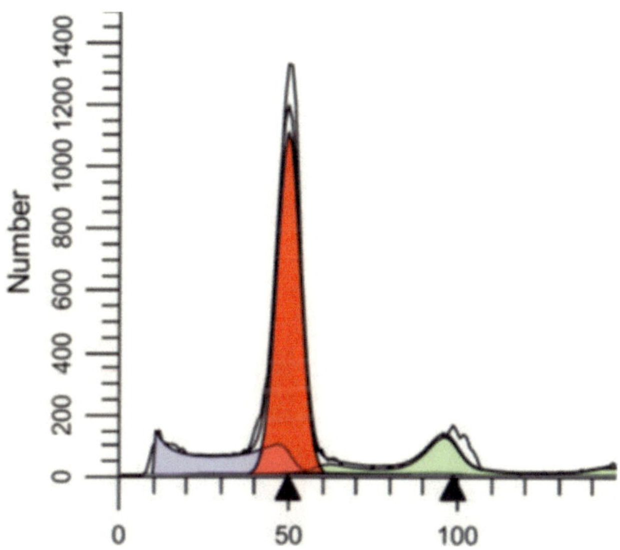

Figure 12.
Aph 6 h after release with AZD in release medium.

incubation. These further studies may provide evidence as to why the longer iron depletion affects synthesis of cell cycle related proteins. These studies should initially put an emphasis on inhibition of promoters (i.e., E2F isoforms, or NFR2, etc., see below).

2.1 Selected iron associated cell death and the oxidative state

Until 10 years ago programed cell death with a specific DNA "ladder" measured on gels, particularly in cancer cells, was ascribed to a process called apoptosis [29, 30]. Evidence for apoptosis was often used to validate anti-neoplastic agents studied *in vitro*. Further studies later showed that apoptosis associated with cells treated with cancer chemotherapeutic agents, or a normal process such as depletion of

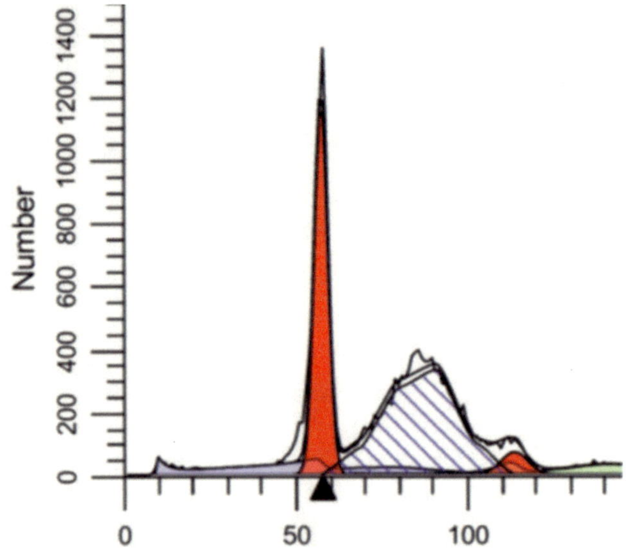

Figure 13.
HU at time of release.

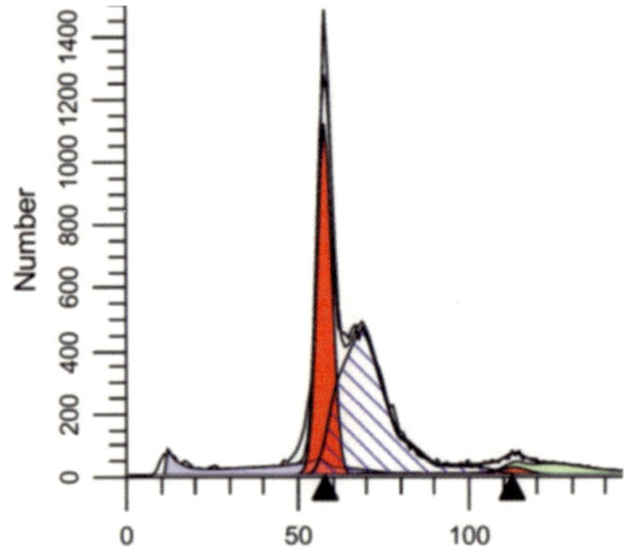

Figure 14.
Six hours after release in medium with no addition.

specific antibody producing B cells, apoptosis was mainly described as a caspase-dependent process [31]. Recently, several non-apoptotic regulated processes that result in cell death have been discovered [32]. One of these processes has been termed ferroptosis [32]. Ferroptosis is best described as autophagy that results in cell death, or autophagic cell death [32]. Overall this process is a combination of the cell's response to toxicity including but not limited to cancer chemotherapy. When first described, autophagy was deemed a cell's response to toxicity including any toxin, chemotherapeutic insult or even hypoxia [33, 34]. The process was associated with lysosomal degradation of cellular constituents including some organelles [33, 34]. The initiation of autophagy is not thought to be cell cycle specific. Until recently, it was thought to be primarily a protective mechanism by which cells

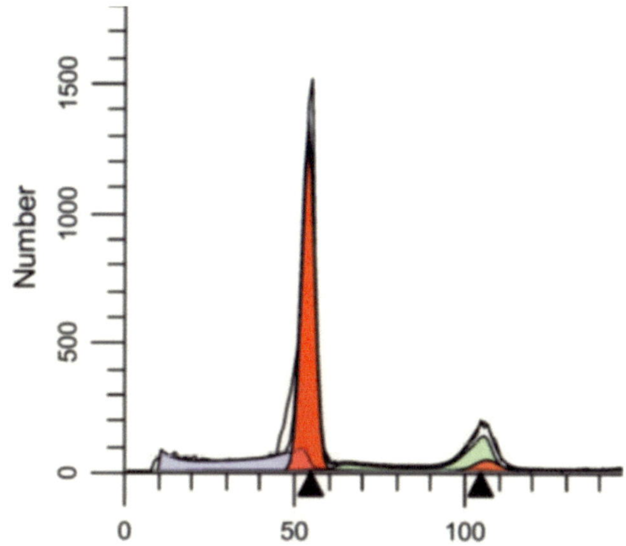

Figure 15.
Aph at time of release with JNJ. JNJ added before release.

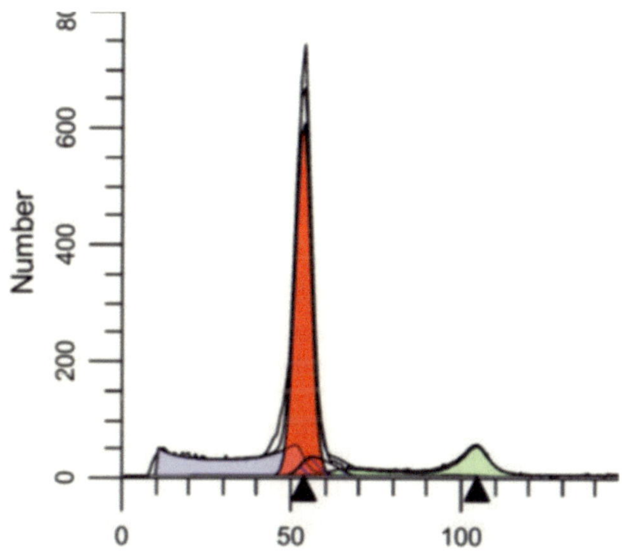

Figure 16.
Six hours after release continued in release medium (no aph).

entered senescence, (arrested in G0/G1 phase), presumably before "start" [35]. This autophagic process was seldom thought to be a cause of cell death. Some have hypothesized that when cancer cells enter senescence a subset become cancer initiating cells, or cancer stem cells resulting in re-emergence of a cancer thought to be in remission [35–37].

Studies have also indicated that senescence associated reprogramming promotes cancer "stemness" that is enriched in relapse tumors [38], resulting in highly aggressive growth potential after escape from G0/G1 cell cycle blockade [38]. Ferroptosis was first described in cancer cells with activation of a common oncogene called RAS [39]. Inappropriate Ras activity results in autonomous cell proliferation. An inhibitor of cell proliferation activated by unregulated RAS was a small molecule called erastin [32, 40]. Erastin was found to increase processes associated with autophagy. By some

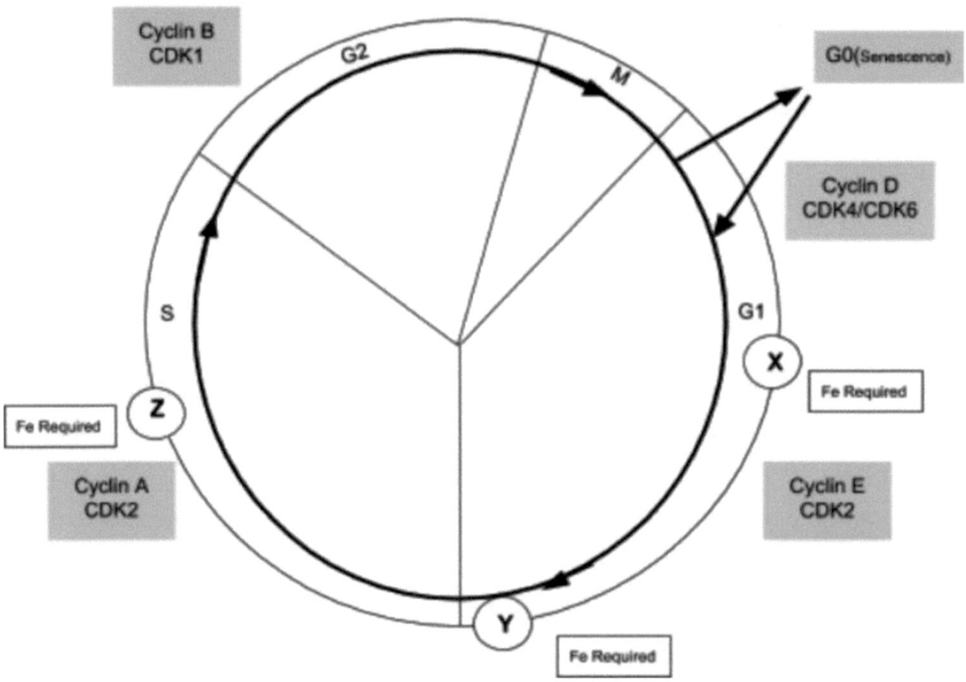

Figure 17.
Simplified cell cycle figure to illustrate steps that require iron. Progression to the next phase requires activation of specific cyclin dependent kinases that depend on binding to each phase specific cyclin(s). X-mid G1 block at least partially caused by iron requirement for psrc activation, Y-putative G1/S block that occurs before DNA synthesis, Z-S phase block at least partly caused by inhibition of RNR. Based on implicating different promoters or changes in the redox state it is quite possible, an iron requirement is necessary in allowing completion of the cell cycle.

accounts [41] increased cellular iron with associated increased reactive oxygen species (ROS) contributed to lipid peroxidation resulting in cell death, thus fulfilling the diagnosis of ferroptosis. In certain instances initiation of this process can influence some neoplastic cells to become more sensitive to chemotherapy [42, 43]. The process may also be accelerated by a decrease in ferroportin [44], the only protein that promotes cellular iron efflux, resulting in a net increase in cellular bioavailable iron [45]. Therefore, the use of passive iron chelation (such as DFO) may actually protect certain proliferating cells from autophagy during cell cycle arrest. This process may be of benefit for normal cells during proliferation [46, 47], but disadvantageous for certain cancer cells during treatment.

Although the precise definition of ferroptosis requires evidence for autophagic cell death, in some instances apoptosis may also be part of the process [48]. Some studies suggest lysosomal leak degrades ferritin, releasing ferritin iron that stimulates lipid peroxidation and is associated with changes of autophagy that can lead to cell death [49]. More recently, p53 has been identified as a ferroptosis inducer by inhibiting cystine uptake, decreasing the cells ability to counteract oxidative processes possibly via decreased GSH, resulting in increased cellular ROS and sensitivity to ferroptosis. Less reducing potential, such as erastin's mechanism of action, was thought to be the main cause of differences in the oxidative state among cell types, but iron concentration and/or iron distribution also plays a part. The p53 effect is thought to be metabolic in nature and not directly related to p53 effects on cell cycle, but it has stimulated interest in novel anticancer agents [50, 51]. It is quite possible that more efficient lipid soluble iron chelators may be more effective in promoting cell death from autophagy due to processes associated with ferroptosis such as lipid peroxidation.

For example, a recent study has shown that polyamines via several pathways are involved with cancer cell proliferation, and these polyamine pathways are stimulated by iron. Thus, specific iron chelation not only inhibits cell growth by mechanisms detailed above, but also inhibits the cellular proliferation caused by the stimulating effect of activated polyamines [52]. Another study has shown that increasing levels of the CDK inhibitor p21 are associated with iron chelation [27], which can have variable effects on inhibition of cell growth depending on the type of chelator as well as the cell type [53]. The study that emphasizes some of these concepts, from the laboratory of DR Richardson, involves "targeting" oncogenic nuclear factor kappa B signaling [54] with redox-active agents. Under normal conditions nuclear factor kappa B signaling occurs under different immunologic conditions [55]. However, aberrant activation of this pathway results in tumorigenesis and unregulated cancer cell proliferation. A hypothesis advanced is the use of lipophilic thiosemicarbazone chelators, first studied extensively in 2006 as having potent antitumor activity, that could potentially overcome resistance to chemotherapeutics [56]. The new studies [54, 57] detail that thiosemicarbazones "form redox-active metal complexes that generate high ROS levels." It is explained that nuclear factor kappa B signaling is actually activated when ROS is in sub-lethal amounts. However, higher ROS generation will inhibit this signaling as one adjunct toward cancer cell death, as opposed to lower ROS generation leading to autophagy, leading to cellular senescence with resistance to anticancer therapy and possible tumor progression. Cell death (ferroptosis) as opposed to autophagic senescence can depend on the tissue type, the redox state, the dose of the lipophilic chelator used and the amount of bioavailable iron.

In recent studies now in press we found that in genomic studies of acute myelogenous leukemia (AML) patients that had low ferroportin message had significantly improved survival compared to those in the higher message group. Using AML cell lines and AML patient derived cells we confirmed that low ferroportin expression compared with high expression resulted in greater iron uptake, faster rates of proliferation, and more sensitivity to chemotherapy. At least in AML where survival is dependent on chemotherapy response higher rates of cellular iron incorporation may improve survival [58].

3. Conclusion

Iron deficiency caused by chelation has been shown to inhibit cellular proliferation, particularly in rapidly growing cancer cells *in vitro* since the 1970s. Since then, iron depletion has been shown to block specific cell cycle processes associated with events in G1, S and probably the G1/S phase transition. Clinical studies of iron depletion have supported many of these findings, and a few select investigational clinical agents that interfere with iron or deplete cells of iron have been utilized in cancer chemotherapy studies. Data are presented regarding specific cell cycle events associated with iron depletion, and some differences in these events among different cell types are described. Passive iron chelation may better pinpoint a step in the metabolic or cell proliferation pathways that require iron. Moreover, the concept of ferroptosis associated with excess iron causing autophagic cell death has resulted in a plethora of studies. These investigations have generated renewed interest in lipophilic iron chelators that result in differential iron binding to sub cellular areas based on the malignant cell type. The resulting generation of ROS, inhibition of oncogenic tumor promoters, and associated autophagic cell death (with a certain extent of apoptosis) suggest these compounds might be useful chemotherapeutic agents. In the future, based on differences in neoplastic tissues, a balance between inhibiting cell proliferation by iron depletion and cell death associated with excess iron will require further study to maximize both events using investigational agents. For example, one transcription factor, NRF2, is known for modulating cellular iron homeostasis and is thought to decrease ferroportin in macrophages, presumably as a way to decrease bioavailable and potentially toxic iron in other cells. However, under pathologic conditions, this transcription factor may increase iron retention by malignant cells [59]. Hepcidin, a hormone made in the liver, under normal conditions is stimulated by inflammation and results in degradation of ferroportin in macrophages. This presumably allows for increased storage of iron and lower iron in serum [45]. However, more needs to be known about how hepcidin affects tumor cells under pathologic conditions [45]. In another example it was found that in estrogen receptor positive breast cancer cells, ferroportin message was significantly reduced with estrogen treatment. Of further interest, a functional estrogen response element was identified within a ferroportin promoter that would repress ferroportin expression [60]. Unfortunately, pharmaceutical companies have a protective interest in new agents, especially those that have potential in the lucrative cancer treatment market. Therefore they are hesitant to publish studies showing biologic effects of an agent, particularly if the effect might be construed as leading to a potentially toxic event.

Conflict of interest

There are no conflicts of interest to declare.

Author details

Paul Seligman* and Gamini Siriwardana
School of Medicine, University of Colorado, Aurora, Colorado, USA

*Address all correspondence to: paul.seligman@ucdenver.edu

IntechOpen

© 2019 The Author(s). Licensee IntechOpen. This chapter is distributed under the terms of the Creative Commons Attribution License (http://creativecommons.org/licenses/by/3.0), which permits unrestricted use, distribution, and reproduction in any medium, provided the original work is properly cited.

References

[1] Seligman P, Klausner R, Huebers A. Molecular mechanisms of iron metabolism. In: Molecular Basis of Blood Disease. Neinhaus A, Majerus P, Stamatoyanopoulous G, Leder P editors. Phila: Saunders; 1987:219-244

[2] Bogdan A, Miyazawa M, Hashimoto K, Tsuji Y. Regulators of iron homeostasis: New players in metabolism, cell death and disease. Trends in Biochemical Sciences. 2016;**41**(3):274-286. DOI: 10.1016/j.tibs.2015.11.9012

[3] MacKenzie E. Intracellular iron transport and storage from molecular mechanisms to health implications. Antioxidants & Redox Signaling. 2008;**10**:997-1030

[4] Hentze M, Muckenthaler M, Andrews N. Balancing acts: molecular control of mammalian iron metabolism. Cell. 2004;**117**:285-297

[5] Chitambur C, Massey E, Seligman P. Regulation of transferrin receptor expression on human leukemia cells during proliferation and induction of differentiation. The Journal of Clinical Investigation. 1983;**72**:1314-1325

[6] Seligman P, Crawford E. Treatment of advanced transitional cell carcinoma of the bladder with continuous-infusion gallium nitrate. Journal of the National Cancer Institute. 1991;**83**:1582-1584

[7] Caniglia L. Deferoxamine, cyclophosphamide, etoposide, carboplatin, and thiotepa (D-CeCat): A new cytoreductive chelation-chemotherapy regimen in patients with advanced neuroblastoma. American Journal of Clinical Oncology. 1992;**15**:319-322

[8] Lui GY, Kovacevic Z, Richardson V, Merlot AM, Kalinowski DS, Richardson DR. Targeting cancer by binding iron: Dissecting cellular signaling pathways. Oncotarget. 2015;**6**(22):18748-18779. DOI: 10.18632/oncotarget.4349

[9] Potuckova E, Jansova H, Machacek M, Vavrova A, Haskova P, Tichotova L. Quantitative analysis of the anti-proliferative activity of combinations of selected iron-chelating agents and clinically used anti-neoplastic drugs. PLoS One. 2014;**9**

[10] Chang YC, Lo WJ, Huang YT, Lin CL, Feng CC, Lin HT. Deferasirox has strong anti-leukemia activity but may antagonize the anti-leukemia effect of doxorubicin. Leukemia and Lymphoma. 2017;**58**(9):2176-2184. DOI: 10.1080/10428194.2017.1280604

[11] Pinnix Z, Miller L, Wang R, D'Agostino T, Kute M. Ferroportin and iron regulation in breast cancer progression and prognosis. Science Translational Medicine. 2010;**2**(43):56

[12] Zacharski L, Chow B, Hoes P, Shamayeva G, Baron J, Dalman R. Decreased cancer risk after iron reduction in patients with peripheral arterial disease: results from a randomized trial. Journal of the National Cancer Institute. 2008;**100**:996-1002

[13] Lenarduzzi M, Hui AB, Yue S, Ito E, Shi W, Williams J. Hemochromatosis enhances tumor progression via upregulation of intracellular iron in head and neck cancer. PLoS One. 2013;**8**

[14] Liu X, Lv C, Luan X, Lv M. C282Y polymorphism in the HFE gene is associated with risk of breast cancer. Tumour Biology. 2013;**34**:2759-2764

[15] Hoffbrand A, Ganeshaguru K, Hooton J, Tattersall M. Effect of iron deficiency and deferoxamine on DNA synthesis in human cells. British Journal of Hematology. 1986;**33**:517

[16] Robbins E, Penderson T. Iron: Its intracellular localization and possible role in cell division. Proceedings of the National Academy of Sciences of the United States of America. 1970;**66**:1244

[17] Taetle R, Rhyner K, Castagnola J, Mendelsohn J. Role of transferrin, Fe, and transferrin receptors in myeloid leukemia cell growth. The Journal of Clinical Investigation. 1985;**75**:1061

[18] Hoyes K, Hider R, Porter J. Cell cycle synchronization and growth inhibition by 3-hydroxypyridin-4-one iron chelators in leukemia cell lines. Cancer Research. 1992;**52**:4591-4599

[19] Seguin A, Ward D, Kaplan J. Regulation of ribonucleotide reductase during iron limitation. Molecular Cell. 2011;**44**:683-684

[20] Brodie C, Siriwardana G, Lucas J, Schleicher R, Terada N, Szepesi A. Neuroblastoma sensitivity to growth inhibition by deferrioxamine: Evidence for a block in G1 phase of the cell cycle. Cancer Research. 1993;**53**:3968-3975

[21] Lucas J, Terada N, Szepesi A, Gelfand E. Regulation of synthesis of p34cdc2 and its homologues and their relationship to P110 phosphorylation during cell cycle progression of normal human T cells. Journal of Immunology. 1192;**148**:1804-1811

[22] Blatt J, Stitely S. Antineuroblastoma activity of desferoxamine in human cell lines. Cancer Research. 1987;**47**:1749-1750

[23] Siriwardana G, Seligman P. Two cell cycle blocks caused by iron chelation of neuroblastoma cells: Separating cell cycle events associated with each block. Physiological Reports. 2013;**1**(7):873-885. DOI: 10.1002/phy2.176

[24] Siriwardana G, Seligman P. Iron depletion results in src kinase inhibtion with associated cell cycle arrest in neuroblastoma cells. Physiological Reports. 2015;**3**(3):1123-1132. DOI: 10.14814/phy2.12341

[25] Vazana-Barad L, Granot G, Mor-Tzuntz R, Levi I, Dreyling M, Nathan I, et al. Mechanism of the antitumoral activity of deferasirox, an iron chelation agent, on mantle cell lymphoma. Leukemia and Lymphoma. 2013;**54**(4):851-859. DOI: 10.3109.10428194.2012.734614

[26] Han YH, Moon HJ, You BR, Park WH. The effect of MG 132, a proteasome inhibitor on HeLa cells in relation to cell growth, reactive oxygen species, and GSH. Oncology Reports. 2009;**22**(1):215-221

[27] Fu D, Richardson D. Iron chelation and regulation of the cell cycle: 2 mechanisms of posttranscriptional regulation of the universal cyclin-dependent kinase inhibitor p21C1P1/WAF1 by iron depletion. Blood. 2007;**110**:752-761

[28] Heath E, Bible K, Martell R, Adelman D, LoRusso P. A phase 1 study of SNS-032 (formerly BMS-387032), a potent inhibitor of cyclin-dependent kinases 2, 7 and 9 administered as a single oral dose and weekly infusion in patients with metastatic refractory solid tumors. Investigational New Drugs. 2008;**26**(1):59-65

[29] Lowe S, Lin A. Apoptosis in cancer. Carcinogenesis. 2000;**21**:485-495. DOI: 10.1093/carcin/21.3.485

[30] Elmore S. Apoptosis: A review of programmed cell death. Toxicologic Pathology. 2007;**35**(4):495-516. DOI: 10.1080/01926230701320337

[31] Li J, Yuan J. Caspases in apoptosis and beyond. Oncogene. 2008;**27**: 6194-6206. DOI: 10.1038/onc.2008.297

[32] Dixon S, Lemberg K, Lamprecht M, Skouta R, Zaitesv E, Gleason C, et al.

Ferroptosis: An iron-dependent form of nonapoptotic cell death. Cell. 2012;**149**:1060-1072. DOI: 10.1016/j.cell.2012.03.042

[33] Glick D. Autophagy: Cellular and molecular mechanisms. Journal of Pathology. 2010;**221**(1):3-13. DOI: 10.1002/path.2697

[34] Choi KS. Autophagy and cancer. Experimental and Molecular Medicine. 2012;**44**:109-120

[35] Herranz N, Gil J. Mechanisms and functions of cellular senescence. The Journal of Clinical Investigation. 2018;**128**(4):1238-1246. DOI: 10.1172/JCI95148

[36] Hamai A, Caneque T, Muller S, Mai TT, Hienzsch A, Ginestier C, et al. An iron hand over cancer stem cells. Autophagy. 2017;**14**:1-2. DOI: 10.1080/15548627.2017.1327104

[37] Kondo Y, Kondo S. Autophagy and cancer therapy. Autophagy. 2006;**2**:85-90

[38] Milanovic M, Fan D, Belenki D, Dabritz H, Zhao Z, Yu Y, et al. Senescence-associated reprogramming promotes cancer stemness. Springer Nature. 2018;**553**. DOI: 10.1038/nature25167

[39] Bos JL. Ras oncogenes in human cancer: A review. Cancer Research; 1989;**49**:4682-4689

[40] Lachaier E, Louandre C, Godin C, Saidak Z, Baert M, Diouf M, et al. Sorafenib induces ferroptosis in human cancer cell lines originating from different solid tumors. Anticancer Research. 2014;**34**(11):6417-6422

[41] Ceo JY, Dixon SJ. Mechanisms of Ferroptosis. Cellular and Molecular Life Sciences. 2016;**73**:11-12. DOI: 10.1007/500018-016-2194-1

[42] Yu Y, Xie Y, Cao L, Yang I, Lotze M, Zeh H, et al. The ferroptosis inducer erastic enhances sensitivity of acute myeloid leukemia cells to chemotherapeutic agents. Molecular and Cellular Oncology. 2015;**2**(4). DOI: 10.1080/23723556.2015.1054549

[43] Ma S. Ferroptosis is induced following sinamesine and lapatinib treatment of breast cancer cells. Cell Death & Disease. 2016;**7**:e2307

[44] Geng N, Shi B, Li S, Zhong Z, Li Y, Xua W, et al. Knockdown of ferroportin accelerates erastin-induced ferroptosis in neuroblastoma cells. European Review for Medical and Pharmacological Sciences. 2018;**22**(12):3826-3836. DOI: 10.26355/eurrev_201806_15267

[45] Ward D, Kaplan J. Ferroportin-mediated iron transport: Expression and regulation. Biochim Biophys. 2012;**1823**(9):1426-1433. DOI: 10.1016/j.bbamer.2012.03.004

[46] Moon J, Jeong J, Park S. Deferoxamine inhibits TRAIL-mediated apoptosis via regulation of autophagy in human colon cancer cells. Oncology Reports. 2014;**3**:1171-1176. DOI: 10.3892/or.2014.3676

[47] Kurz T et al. Intralysosomal iron chelation protects against oxidative stress-induced cellular damage. Febs Journal. 2006;**273**:3106-3117. DOI: 10.1111/j.1742-4658.2006.05321.x

[48] Booth L et al. The role of cell signaling in the crosstalk between autophagy and apoptosis. Cell Signaling. 2014;**26**(3):549-558. DOI: 10.1016/j.cellsig.2013.11.028

[49] Yang N et al. Artesunate induces cell death in human cancer cells via enhancing lysosomal function and lysosomal degradation of ferritin. Journal of Biological Chemistry. 2014;**289**(48):33425-33441. DOI: 10.1074/jbcM114.564567

[50] Jiang L et al. Ferroptosis is a p53-mediated activity during tumor

suppression. Nature. 2015;**520**(7545):57-62. DOI: 10.1038/nature14344

[51] Kang R et al. The tumor suppressor protein p53 and the ferroptosis network. Free Radical Biological Medicine. 2018;**18**:50891-55849. DOI: 10.1016/j.freeradbiomed.2018.05.074

[52] Bae D et al. The old and new biochemistry of polyamines. Biochemical and Biophysical Research Communications. 2018;**1862**(9). DOI: 10.1016bbagen2018.6.004

[53] Moussa R, Park K, Kovacevic Z, Richardson D. Ironing out the role of the cyclin-dependent kinase inhibitor, p21 in cancer: Novel iron chelating agents to target p21 expression and activity. Free Radical Biology and Medicine. 2018;**18**:30130-30138. DOI: 10.1016/j.freeradbiomed.2018.03.027

[54] Fouani L, Kovacevic Z, Richardson D. Targeting oncogenic NF-kB signaling with redox-active agents for cancer treatment. Antioxidants and Redox. 2017;**13**:934-942. DOI: 10.1089/ars.2017.7387

[55] Bonizzi G, Karin M. The two NFkB activation pathways and their role in innate and adaptive immunity. 2004;**25**(6):280-288. DOI: 10.1016/j.it.2004.03.008

[56] Whitnall M, Howard J, Ponka P, Richardson D. A class of iron chelators with a wide spectrum of potent antitumor activity that overcomes resistances to chemotherapeutics. Proceedings of the National Academy of Science. 2006;**103**(40):14901-14906. DOI: 10/1073/pnas.0604979103

[57] Fouani L, Kovacevic Z, Richardson D. Targeting oncogenic nuclear factor kappa B signaling with redox-active agents for cancer treatment. Antioxidants and Redox Signaling. 2018;**29**. DOI: 10.1089/ars.2017.7387

[58] Gasparetto M, Pei S, Minhajuddin M, Stevens B, Smith C, Seligman P. Low ferroportin expression in AML is correlated with good risk cytogenetics, improved outcomes and increased sensitivity to chemotherapy. Leukemia Research. May 2019;**80**:1-10. DOI: 10.1016/j.leukres.2019.02.011. [Epub 2019 feb 28]

[59] Kerins M, Ooi A. The roles of NRF2 in modulating cellular iron homeostasis. Antioxidants and Redox Signaling. 10 Dec 2018;**29**(17):1756-1773. DOI: 10.1089/ars.2017.7176

[60] Qian Y, Yin C, Chen Y, Zhang S, Jiang L, Wang F, et al. Estrogen contributes to the regulating iron metabolism through governing ferroptortin signaling via an estrogen response element. Cellular Signaling. 2015;**27**(5):934-942. DOI: 10.1016/j.cellsig.2015.01.017